Helping
Cardiac Patients

*Biobehavioral
and Psychotherapeutic
Approaches*

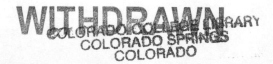

Andrew M. Razin, Ph.D., M.D.

and Associates

Helping
Cardiac Patients

Jossey-Bass Publishers
San Francisco • Washington • London • 1985

HELPING CARDIAC PATIENTS
Biobehavioral and Psychotherapeutic Approaches
by Andrew M. Razin, Ph.D., M.D., and Associates

Library of Congress Cataloging in Publication Data

Razin, Andrew M.
    Helping cardiac patients.

    (A Joint publication in the Jossey-Bass social and
behavioral science series and the Jossey-Bass health
series)
    Includes bibliographies and index.
    1. Cardiovascular system—Diseases—Psychological
aspects. 2. Cardiacs—Rehabilitation. 3. Behavior
modification. I. Title. II. Series: Jossey-Bass
social and behavioral science series. III. Series:
Jossey-Bass health series. [DNLM: 1. Cardiovascular
Diseases—psychology. 2. Cardiovascular Diseases—
therapy. WG 100 R278h]
    RC682.R39   1985   616.1'2'0019   84-47995
    ISBN 0-87589-627-8

Manufactured in the United States of America

The paper in this book meets the guidelines for
permanence and durability of the Committee on
Production Guidelines for Book Longevity of the
Council on Library Resources.

JACKET DESIGN BY WILLI BAUM

FIRST EDITION

Code 8506

A joint publication in
The Jossey-Bass
Social and Behavioral Science Series
and
The Jossey-Bass Health Series

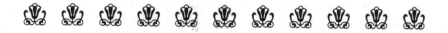

Foreword

Only in the last century have human diseases been defined primarily in biological terms. Medical technology has led to an exponential expansion of our knowledge about the physical aspects of health and illness, reinforcing the pathologist Rudolf Virchow's statement "Disease has its origin in the disease of the cell." Throughout this time, however, a few physicians—beginning with Johann Christian Heinroth, Maximilian Jacobi, and Sigmund Freud—struggled to retain a more comprehensive, "psychosomatic" concept of health and disease, to include psychological and environmental phenomena in the etiology and definition of medical illnesses. Most recently George Engel has been the leading spokesperson for this position, which he terms the "biopsychosocial model." This, the most current label for the quite ancient view of human disease, implies the complex interaction of biological and mental phenomena within the organism, which is also openly interacting with its environment.

Of all biological systems, the cardiovascular has been most clearly recognized as influenced by psychological factors. John Hunter, the anatomist and surgeon, has been quoted as saying, "My life is in the hands of any rascal who chooses to anger me," apparently referring to his high blood pressure.

William Sweetser cited the common knowledge of physicians in the mid-nineteenth century when he wrote, "Under the sudden shock of grief, the heart and nervous system may become so greatly agitated and disturbed as to place the life of the individual in much peril." Flanders Dunbar in the 1930s and 1940s identified personality profiles of patients with a variety of cardiovascular disorders. Many of these characteristics are similar to the more recent observations and formulations of Meyer Friedman and Ray Rosenman in the 1950s and 1960s, who popularized a behavior pattern, called "Type A," which is associated with coronary artery disease. Indeed, this connection between behavior and a particular medical illness was perhaps the first such relationship generally accepted by medicine in at least a hundred years.

Despite some progress in the acceptance of the importance of psychosocial factors in medical disease, the struggle with the "biomedical model" continues. In the Virchow tradition, modern medicine still attempts to define disease simplistically, as a biological process with a unitary and linear causation. The less tangible psychological and social phenomena continue to be ignored whenever possible. For example, coronary artery bypass grafting (CABG) continues to increase in frequency and cost, despite its questionable effectiveness in promoting lengthened survival or successful vocational rehabilitation. The effectiveness rate of CABG in pain relief is actually similar to that achieved by several previous treatment methods, which were then shown to have no major biological effects, despite providing good to excellent relief of angina.

The chapters in this book cover four major aspects of cardiovascular disease in which behavioral, psychological, interpersonal, and environmental factors are important in etiology and/or management. This material is important in its own right because of the high frequency of cardiovascular disease. There is an added significance in this work, however, because research in the psychosocial aspects of other medical illnesses is not as far advanced as that presented in this volume. These highly developed studies can serve as inspirations and models for research in diseases involving other biological systems. For example, cardiac pathogenicity, which was broadly attributed to a somewhat heterogeneous "Type A" behavior pattern, has now been more specifically attributed to difficulties in handling anger, which is but one of several components of the Type A pattern. This suggests the importance of defining specific coping styles and their effectiveness in other diseases, rather than overall character traits. As we pursue the "mysterious leap" from mental to biological phenomena, the extensive knowledge and advances cited in this volume should stand as a testimony to the distances the field has come and also has yet to go.

January 1985   F. Patrick McKegney, M.D.
        Professor of Psychiatry
        Chief, Division of
        Consultation-Liaison Psychiatry
        Albert Einstein College of Medicine/
        Montefiore Medical Center

To Hilary, Elizabeth, and Kathryn,
with all my love

Preface

Over the past two decades, there has been growing interest among clinicians and researchers in psychological aspects of heart disease. Thus, psychosocial factors in the etiology of hypertension and arrhythmias, the role of Type A behavior in coronary artery disease, psychological factors in postoperative cardiac recovery, the use of behavioral techniques in the control of arrhythmias and hypertension, and the use of group therapy following myocardial infarction have all gained increasing recognition.

The growth of interest and knowledge in this area is reflected in a growing literature. To date, however, there has been no comprehensive attempt to integrate this work for clinicians and researchers. This volume synthesizes for the first time the clinical and research literature on various biobehavioral and psychotherapeutic interventions in four major cardiovascular problems. We use the terms "biobehavioral" and "psychotherapeutic" to refer to a broad range of interventions—from traditional psychodynamic psychotherapy, through various behavioral and didactic methods, to psychopharmacological and environmental manipulations. Similarly, the range of literature is also broad, encompassing not only rigorous, methodologically sound research but also anecdotal reports and clinical lore. Finally, our intended audience should be broad. While we have addressed this work primarily to clinicians (of all psychotherapeutic disciplines), we hope that researchers and teachers, as well as certain nonpsychiatric medical and nursing staff (such as directors of coronary care units and cardiac nurse-practitioners), will also find the book relevant to their clinical work.

Each of the four cardiac problems in which biobehavioral and psychotherapeutic interventions have most commonly been attempted is represented by a chapter in this volume: hypertension, cardiac surgery, arrhythmias, and coronary artery disease.

In their chapter on hypertension, James J. Lynch and Sue Ann Thomas critically reconsider some common assumptions and conceptualizations underlying the behavioral interventions (conditioning and biofeedback) used in hypertension. In fact, their critique seems applicable to behavioral medical interventions in general and thus warrants close scrutiny. They then describe a potentially significant discovery: the hypertensive effects of speaking. Their own intervention program, transactional psychophysiology, which takes into account this effect, might appear in some ways similar to usual biofeedback; yet it is different in several respects, including its use of psychodynamic interpretation and confrontations. Thus, the work and the viewpoint of these authors are exciting and possibly revolutionary for both psychophysiological theory and clinical practice.

Cardiac arrhythmias are considered by Michael Feuerstein and Ronald A. Cohen. Their detailed yet lucid description of normal and pathological cardiac electrical activity should enable both physicians and nonphysicians to appreciate the biopsychosocial complexity and clinical heterogeneity in this group of disorders. They also provide a comprehensive, critical review of interventions in these disorders. The reader will quickly realize that here, as with hypertension, the vast majority of reported interventions have been behavioral. Finally, the authors delineate their own biobehavioral diagnostic and therapeutic approach, offering examples of cases and instruments from their clinical work.

A variety of cardiac conditions, including coronary artery disease, valvular disease, and arrhythmias, may be treated surgically. Thus, the chapter by Larry S. Goldman and Chase Patterson Kimball, like the others, also deals with a heterogeneous group of disorders. The authors discuss the implications of preoperative (screening/predictive) psychological patient assessments, they review attempts at preoperative and postoperative intervention, and they provide vivid descriptions of patients' subjective experiences pre- and postoperatively. In particular, they present a comprehensive and clinically instructive understanding of the phenomenon known as postcardiotomy psychosis, or "ICU psychosis."

Andrew M. Razin's chapter first acquaints the reader with the pathology and pathophysiology of coronary artery disease. As with the other disorders, the heterogeneity of this apparently homogeneous group of disorders becomes abundantly clear. Razin goes on to review critically the psychosocial interventions aimed at prevention, postsurgical care, and rehabilitation. Particular emphasis is given to Type A behavior and some of the promising attempts to modify it and also to postmyocardial infarction psychotherapies, individual and group. Razin draws on both research and clinical experience in offering clinicians guidelines for working with myocardial infarction patients and their families. He also provides guidelines for work with "cardiac neurotic" and angina patients.

As all four chapters make clear, there have been great advances over the past few decades in basic cardiac physiology, improved understanding of etiological (risk) factors, improved medical and surgical treatments, and the development of biobehavioral and psychotherapeutic interventions for cardiac disorders. Yet it is equally clear that we are quite some distance from being able to prescribe specific, individually relevant therapeutic interventions that are empirically supported. With certain notable exceptions, perhaps most clearly the areas of hypertension, some arrhythmias, and Type A behavior, much of our literature is clinical lore—immensely valuable, to be sure, but very much in need of systematic assessment if this body of work is to constitute a lasting contribution. It is therefore our hope not only to provide the large body of clinicians with useful guidelines but also to inspire perhaps a few to evaluate systematically some portion of this cumulated body of clinical knowledge.

Bronx, New York   Andrew M. Razin, Ph.D., M.D.
January 1985

Contents

The Authors

Andrew M. Razin, Ph.D., M.D., is director of the Psychiatric Consultation-Liaison Service at North Central Bronx Hospital (Albert Einstein College of Medicine). There he is actively involved in the teaching and practice of psychosocial aspects of rehabilitation and prevention in cardiac disease and other disorders. His clinical work emphasizes interdisciplinary, interspecialty biopsychosocial approaches to the treatment of the medically ill.

Razin received his B.A. degree from Brown University (1967) and his Ph.D. degree (1972) from Columbia University. Following a two-year postdoctoral fellowship at the Yale University School of Medicine, he attended the Albert Einstein College of Medicine, where he received the Rock-Sleyster Award in psychiatry and his M.D. degree (1976). Razin then completed his psychiatric residency at Einstein, during which he served as chief resident and was designated a Laughlin Fellow by the American College of Psychiatrists. Following residency, he joined the faculty at Albert Einstein, where he has since served as assistant clinical professor in the Department of Psychiatry. His research interests originally focused on the outcome and process of psychotherapy, especially psychotherapist factors. He has published widely on these issues in psychology and psychiatry journals. In particular, the volume *Effective Psychotherapy: A Handbook of Research* (1977), which he co-edited and contributed to, treats nearly two dozen psychotherapist factors and their relationships to process and outcome. After his medical training, Razin's research interests expanded to include psychotherapeutic intervention in cardiovascular disease, and in particular the modification of behavioral cardiac risk factors, such as Type A behavior.

Ronald A. Cohen, Ph.D., is assistant professor, Department of Neurology, University of Massachusetts Medical Center, Worcester.

Michael Feuerstein, Ph.D., is associate professor, Department of Psychiatry, and director, Behavior Therapy Programs, Division of Behavioral and Psychosocial Medicine, University of Rochester School of Medicine.

Larry S. Goldman, M.D., is assistant professor, Department of Psychiatry, University of Chicago School of Medicine.

Chase Patterson Kimball, M.D., is professor of psychiatry and medicine, Division of Biological Sciences, University of Chicago Pritzker School of Medicine; professor in the College (Behavioral Sciences), University of Chicago; and director, Psychiatric Liaison-Consultation Service, University of Chicago Hospitals and Clinics.

James J. Lynch, Ph.D., is professor of psychology, University of Maryland, and director, Psychophysiological Clinic, University of Maryland School of Medicine.

Sue Ann Thomas, R.N., Ph.D., is assistant professor, School of Nursing, University of Maryland, and clinical director, Psychophysiological Clinic, University of Maryland School of Medicine.

Helping
Cardiac Patients

*Biobehavioral
and Psychotherapeutic
Approaches*

1

Hypertension: Controlling Blood Pressure

James J. Lynch, Ph.D.
Sue Ann Thomas, R.N., Ph.D.

The past few years have witnessed a sharp increase in interest in nonpharmacological treatment approaches to essential hypertension. There is increasing evidence that nondrug alternatives can be effective in lowering blood pressure (Shapiro and Goldstein, 1982; Seer, 1979; Shapiro and others, 1977); that standard drug treatments can produce undesirable side effects, including depression, insomnia, impotency, and generalized lethargy (Sterling and Eyer, 1981); and that some drugs can exacerbate rather than ameliorate certain cardiovascular problems (Duke, 1978; Ames and Hill, 1976; Holland and others, 1981; Hollifield and Slaton, 1981). The most obvious drug management problems with hypertension, however, involve compliance with medication regimens: "There are 26 million individuals who are aware of elevated blood pressures but whose condition remains either

1

untreated or inadequately controlled. . . . Either they have been noncompliant with recommendations to seek therapy (14 million individuals) or they have been noncompliant with therapeutic recommendations (12 million)" (Reichgott and Simons-Morton, 1983, p. 21). This group represents at least 44 percent of all hypertensive individuals. Among the more troubling aspects of drug compliance is the fact that those who have more severe forms of the disease (increased symptoms and increased disability) do not show better compliance. Indeed, those who have taken medicines for over five years tend to comply less with drug regimens than those more recently diagnosed (Reichgott and Simons-Morton, 1983). In addition, several widely used antihypertensive agents (such as Clonidine, Quanabenz, and beta blockers) can cause serious rebound hypertensive and cardiac effects if the patient abruptly stops the medications—a problem frequently occurring with drug noncompliance.

Moreover, although drugs can reduce the overall mortality from stroke and from renal and heart failure in patients with moderate hypertension (those with diastolic pressures between 105 and 120 mm Hg), similar therapeutic benefits have not been shown yet with mild or borderline hypertensives (those with diastolic pressures between 90 and 105 mm Hg) (United States Public Health Service Hospitals Cooperative Study Group, 1972; Veterans Administration Cooperative Study Group, 1967, 1970, 1972; Smith, Johnson, and Bromer, 1975). A large-scale epidemiological study, the Multiple Risk Factor Intervention Trial (MRFIT), found a higher incidence of mortality in that group of mild hypertensives who had electrocardiographic abnormalities and who were treated with antihypertensive medicines than in those who were not treated with medicines (Multiple Risk Factor Intervention Trial Research Group, 1982). Evidence from this study, as well as a growing literature on the therapeutic benefits of more benign nonpharmacological treatment approaches, has led the Food and Drug Administration to recommend that physicians should "initiate treatment of mild blood pressure, particularly in the range of 90-94 mm Hg diastolic pressure, *with nonpharmacological measures* as long as this treatment is effective in maintaining blood pressure" (Brandt, 1983).

In this chapter we will briefly review the major nonpharmacological treatment approaches for hypertension and address some of the issues raised by these approaches. We will also describe a new approach that we have developed—transactional psychophysiology. Certain nonpharmacological factors that influence blood pressure (BP)—factors such as cigarette smoking, obesity, dysfunctional dietary habits, and lack of exercise—will not be reviewed. Each of these living habits has well-known influences on the cardiovascular system, as well as well-known psychological and behavioral components that can influence BP. It is, however, widely accepted that any systematic treatment of hypertension—whether pharmacological, psychological, behavioral, or interpersonal—would logically recommend changes in the health habits of daily life (no smoking, a balanced diet, weight loss, and regular dynamic exercise).

The Mosaic Theory of Hypertension

Sterling and Eyer (1981, p. 18) have observed that basically only three physiological possibilities exist for raising BP: "The body can (1) increase the amount of salt water in the vascular system (by action of the kidney); (2) decrease the volume of the vascular system (by constriction of vessels); (3) increase the rate at which fluid is pumped through the system (by increasing output of the heart)." This description succinctly summarizes the well-known physiological formula that Blood Pressure = Peripheral Resistance X Cardiac Output (where Cardiac Output equals Stroke Volume X Heart Rate).

While this formula theoretically ought to make it relatively easy to identify and assign weights to the various physiological factors that contribute to sustained elevated BP, the fact is that in only 10-15 percent of all cases can a precise physiological source for the problem be identified. In the remaining 85-90 percent of cases, the cause cannot be attributed to any specific pathophysiology (Kaplan, 1980). And although the major components of the equation have been clearly identified, research investigators differ widely on the relative importance of various physiological and neurochemical factors that can influence each of these components (Sterling and Eyer,

1981). Not only do sharp differences exist in this regard, but variables such as heredity, predisposition to salt intake, obesity, and abnormalities in the renin-angiotensin system also can co-vary or interact with the cardiovascular system in a number of different ways. For example, obesity can alter BP directly by altering the hemodynamic load placed on the cardiovascular sys-tem. At the same time, obesity can also distort body image and one's sense of identity and well-being, and thus contribute to serious psychological stress, especially in interpersonal interac-tions, which can also significantly increase the work of the cardiovascular system. As we shall see, these two variables—in-creased hemodynamic load and disturbance in body image—can also independently, additively, or interactively act to alter BP elevations during human communications. Thus, a single physi-cal factor, obesity, can influence the cardiovascular system in a variety of ways.

Irwin Page (see Weiner, 1979, p. 40) has described as-pects of this complex reality in his mosaic theory of hyperten-sion: "Hypertension under this concept can begin in many ways and also develop in many ways. . . . The theory does not rule out the initiation of hypertension by one stimulus. Experience, however, shows that what appears to be one stimulus usually in-volves multiple mechanisms ranging from genetic to emotional stress." Agreeing with this conceptual framework, Weiner has similarly noted that elevations in BP most likely result from an interaction of a variety of physiological, genetic, psychological, environmental, social, economic, and family factors.

While hypertension itself is a significant predictor of who will subsequently develop other cardiovascular diseases, such as stroke, congestive heart failure, and coronary heart disease, there are no comparable predictors of who will become hyper-tensive (Kesteloot and Joossens, 1980). Furthermore, those sets of physiological factors that contribute to transient elevations in BP need not be the same ones that maintain chronic levels of elevated BP. Given the potential complex etiology for the prob-lem, it seems highly unlikely that any single simple set protocol —whether pharmacological or nonpharmacological—would be universally successful in lowering BP in all hypertensive individuals. Indeed, as we shall see, evidence suggests that a mosaic treatment approach which we call transactional psychophysiology (TP) may be the best approach to a disease that is most likely mosaic in its origins.

Set and Setting Variables in Blood Pressure Assessment

In addition to the complex etiology of hypertension, a number of set and setting variables have likewise contributed to differences in BP readings, thus rendering interpretations of both pharmacological and nonpharmacological treatments alike quite problematic. One such set and setting factor is embedded in the very methods used to detect BP. The traditional method of taking BP with a stethoscope (the auscultatory method) is well known to have the potential to alter BP (Wolf and others, 1955). In addition, nonspecific factors surrounding the measurement procedure—factors such as home setting, clinic, or workplace; status, sex, and racial differences; and the significance attached to the reading itself (if it is taken, for example, for insurance screening)—can also alter pressure readings significantly.

The recent development of automatic noninvasive computerized methods to assess BP has revealed another dimension to set and setting variables that previously had gone unrecognized. That is, the mere act of speaking can contribute to rapid and significant elevations in BP, with decrease back to baseline levels soon after a person is quiet once again (Lynch and others, 1980). This response has been consistently observed in populations that range from schoolchildren (Thomas and others, 1984a) to geriatric patients, and from normotensive to severely hypertensive individuals (Lynch and others, 1982a), and in patients who have been medicated with antihypertensive agents (Lynch and others, 1981). The magnitude of the BP rise during speech is influenced by the rate of speech (Friedmann and others, 1982), audience size (Thomas and others, 1984b), status differences (Long and others, 1982), environmental setting (Pickering and others, 1982b), and baseline BP (Lynch and others, 1981).

This previously unrecognized direct influence of speaking

could have a major impact on the determination of resting BP and makes it difficult to interpret previous normative studies on hypertension that did not control for this problem. While silence is structurally built into the auscultatory BP measurement procedure, it now seems clear that who is speaking just before pressure is measured can have a significant influence on the reading. If the patient speaks, BP may be higher than normal; if the physician talks and the patient listens intently, BP could very well fall below its normal baseline levels. Since the auscultatory measurement procedure is inherently social in nature, it is highly unlikely that both the physician and patient will remain quiet just before the measurement itself. These links between speaking and BP unfortunately cast serious doubt on the BP norms used in epidemiological studies on which much of our current knowledge of hypertension is based. They also pose very real problems for the evaluation of outcome measures for the various pharmacological and nonpharmacological approaches aimed at lowering BP.

The entire question of establishing norms for true baseline measures of BP is only now being given more concentrated attention with the development of twenty-four-hour ambulatory measurement protocols. Pickering, Harshfield, and their associates (Harshfield and others, 1982; Pickering and others, 1982a, 1982b) have recently shown that pressures measured casually in the clinic do not accurately reflect average twenty-four-hour pressures. A blood pressure taken in the setting of a physician's office for the evaluation of high BP may be artificially elevated and not representative of the baseline pressure. Conversely, ambulatory blood pressures represent a large number of measurements made throughout the day and so are potentially more representative of a patient's cardiovascular load. In light of the emergence of twenty-four-hour recordings of blood pressure, it would seem that coding of specific interpersonal interactions, especially when the person is speaking, would enhance understanding of the data obtained. A notable example in this regard are the reports by Pickering and his associates (1982a, 1982b) at Cornell Medical School. They found that a variety of social interactions, such as talking on the telephone, were linked to extremely high ambulatory readings of BP.

Cardiovascular Correlates of Fight/Flight

Regardless of the methodological problems in BP assessment, and the wide variety of potential factors contributing to pressure elevations, and the various treatment modalities used to lower it, certain assumptions about BP regulation are widely shared, especially in nonpharmacological treatment approaches. These assumptions concern the links between emotional arousal and BP elevations, and their origins can be traced back to the pioneering studies of Walter Cannon (1929). Early in the twentieth century, Cannon demonstrated that emotional arousal elicits a variety of autonomic nervous system reactions, which he called the "fight-or-flight" response. This generalized autonomic bodily mobilization involves activation of various neurohumoral, endocrine, cardiovascular, skeletal muscular, and respiratory factors. In Cannon's view, rapid increases in blood pressure, heart rate, and blood flow, as well as alterations in neuroendocrine function, are physiological responses that prepare an animal to fight or run away; when the animal is calmed (through petting or gentle reassurance), these autonomically mediated fight/flight reactions decrease rapidly. While details of Cannon's fight/flight response have been greatly expanded in the intervening years, the fundamental outlines of his theoretical assumptions about links between emotional arousal and BP changes have remained intact.

An important extension of Cannon's notions about fight/ flight was added at virtually the same time by Ivan P. Pavlov (1927). Pavlov's theoretical interests, like those of Cannon, were rooted in the concept of homeostasis. He originally set out to delineate the various homeostatic reflex mechanisms involved in one component of the autonomic nervous system—namely, the digestive system. As his research continued, however, Pavlov realized that internal physiological reflexes had to keep themselves in balance with a constantly changing external environment. He proposed that there are two types of reflexes: uncon-

ditional reflexes, which maintain homeostasis in the internal milieu; and conditional reflexes, which maintain homeostatic balance with the external world. Thus, Pavlov added a new dimension to the concept of homeostasis, one that explained how
animals keep their physiological systems in balance in the face
of a constantly changing external world. Just as unconditional
stimuli (such as food, pain, noise, or biochemical shifts in the
body) elicit unconditional reflexes inside the body (including
cardiovascular changes), conditional stimuli can elicit conditional responses. Pavlov was the first to indicate how reflex
physiology operates to regulate an animal's heart and blood
pressure, not only in response to various internal homeostatic
demands but also in response to various symbolic stimuli in an
animal's external world. He extended Cannon's idea of fight/
flight to include not only an animal's autonomic reactions to a
perceived threat but also conditional reflex reactions to symbolic stimuli that had been paired with threats in the past.

   Pavlov and Cannon had made empirical observations of
transient arousals of the autonomic nervous system. Later investigators assumed that these transient changes observed in the
fight/flight response (both unconditional and conditional) could
be generalized to incorporate a broad range of more prolonged
changes that were involved in psychosomatic or psychophysiological disease. Clinical problems such as hypertension were seen
within this conceptual framework as manifestations of a more
chronic or continuous physiological state of hypervigilance or
continuous state of fight/flight. The belief that rapid elevations
in BP are part of a generalized fight/flight response led to a variety of attempts to use nonpharmacological methods to control
hypertension. If emotional arousal had contributed to the disease, it was argued, then techniques that lower emotional arousal
should be beneficial in lowering BP.

   While the dynamic foundations of Pavlov's theories were
rooted in the concept of homeostasis and reflex physiology,
psychologists and behavioral scientists unfortunately presumed
that he was describing quite another phenomenon, one that involved a form of learning related to the conditioning principles
established by investigators such as Thorndike and Watson

(Lynch, 1970). These investigators tended to regard learning or behavior as a unitary phenomenon, whereas Pavlov was concerned with the reflex wiring of specific organs. Pavlov himself believed that the specific conditional reflexes of individual organ systems were wired to change quickly as environmental conditions changed. Otherwise, as he pointed out, conditional reflex mechanisms would quickly become maladaptive and serve no fundamental homeostatic function. Thus, he used the terms "conditional reflex" and "conditional response" to imply that these various physiological reflexes quickly accommodate to changes in environmental conditions. Ironically, though, his core terms were mistranslated as conditioned reflex and conditioned response—leading many to presume that he was describing a more global, unitary type of learning rather than the conditioning of specific organ system reflexes (Pavlov, 1932; Gantt, 1967a, 1967b). Psychologists and behavioral scientists interested in learning theory incorrectly deduced that Pavlov was describing learning that was more or less established in a unified manner.

Pavlov empirically addressed the question of how environment interacts with reflex physiology; thus, he was the first to provide a conceptual framework to help explain how the environment can homeostatically influence systems such as BP. Unfortunately, the fundamental blurring of certain aspects of his key ideas led many behavioral scientists to think that a set of fixed environmental manipulations could be used to lower BP and that these manipulations would then subsequently keep it constant once the "learning" had occurred.

In spite of this general problem, others clearly understood the central thread of his model. The cardiovascular correlates of Pavlovian conditional reactions have been systematically explored by a number of researchers (Gantt, 1960, 1967a, 1967b; Gantt and Hoffman, 1940; Obrist, 1976; Obrist and others, 1970, 1972, 1974, 1978, 1979; Rescorla and Solomon, 1967; Dykman, Gantt, and Whitehorn, 1956; Smith and Stebbins, 1965; Cohen, 1974). Gantt in particular, a physician who had worked directly with Pavlov for seven years, was the first to measure the cardiovascular correlates of Pavlovian conditional reflexes. By monitoring the cardiovascular components of various conditional reflexes, he added an important dimension to the conceptual framework of his teacher. Gantt observed that the various bodily systems could exhibit markedly different patterns of conditional reflex formation. He found, for example, that just one pairing of a tone with a shock to the forelimb of a dog was sufficient to elicit marked heart rate and BP conditional reflex increases, even though the skeletal muscle components of the reflex (that is, conditional flexion of the paw) usually took many pairings of the tone and shock before the conditional flexion appeared. By contrast, during extinction (that is, when the tone was presented repeatedly without the electric shock) he observed that the somatic conditional reflexes would quickly disappear, while the cardiovascular conditional reactions could continue for thousands of trials. In some dogs the cardiovascular conditional reactions actually became exaggerated after the conditional signal was no longer paired with shock. Gantt (1944) labeled the phenomenon schizokinesis, or a split in the development and extinction of visceral and somatic conditional reflexes.

Gantt's observations suggested that cardiovascular concomitants of Pavlovian fight/flight conditional responses could be conditioned far more rapidly than the somatic components, but once established the cardiovascular reactions were very difficult to eliminate (Gantt, 1967a, 1967b). In a very real sense, his work pointed out how Pavlovian conditional reflexes, which were initially part and parcel of an overall adaptive response to fight/flight, could become maladaptive reactions, autonomic conditional responses that continued long after the real threat had been eliminated. His observations helped support the idea that early conditioning is especially crucial for the overall regulation of the cardiovascular system. They suggested that humans could react to long-forgotten associations with increases in their heart rate and BP, even though all external somatic conditional reactions had long since disappeared. That is, conditional stimuli associated with early traumatic experiences could elicit conditional cardiovascular fight/flight reactions years after the external threat had been eliminated. Subsequently, Obrist and his colleagues developed the links between the somatic and cardiovascular system and Pavlovian conditioning into a comprehensive theory. Their work has provided an important conceptual framework linking adaptive and maladaptive cardiovascular functioning to behavior (Obrist, 1976; Obrist and others, 1970, 1972, 1974, 1978, 1979).

Psychotherapy as a Treatment for Hypertension

The pioneering physiological studies of Pavlov and Cannon were conducted at virtually the same time that Sigmund Freud outlined his psychodynamic formulations about human personality. Freud believed that human personality involves a rather fixed set of psychodynamic variables, including ego defenses, that are profoundly shaped by early developmental experiences. As such, his conceptual point of view complemented the theoretical frame of reference of Pavlov and Cannon. In a Freudian context, Pavlov's visceral conditional responses could be seen in human beings as reactions superimposed on a biological system that had been structurally set, by personality, to respond in a stereotypical fashion much earlier in life. The crucial difference between the two approaches is that Freud focused on the interpersonal domain of early experience and on the crucial significance of primary objects (the child's parents) as determining subsequent emotional reactivity.

The first efforts to integrate Freudian thinking with the physiological observations of Cannon and Pavlov in terms of hypertension were made by Franz Alexander. In the mid-1930s Alexander began to investigate the personality and psychodynamics of hypertensive patients. When he began his studies, no effective pharmacological remedies for hypertension existed, and so he hoped to ascertain whether psychodynamically oriented insight psychotherapy could be used to help patients lower their blood pressure. Extending Cannon's fight/flight response into the domain of personality theory, Alexander hypothesized that chronic BP elevations are caused by more enduring personality characteristics of hypertensive patients. He theorized that a specific cluster of personality traits may lead certain individuals to maintain a chronic hypertensive state of fight/flight. His assumptions were grounded in Cannon's discoveries of the links between emotional arousal, fight/flight, and the overall regulation of BP, as well as in Pavlov's evidence that such reactions can be elicited by symbolic or conditional signals paired with danger in the past. If hypertensive patients could gain insight about the dynamic conflicts that led them to maintain a state of chronic hypervigilance, Alexander hypothesized, they might be able to learn more adaptive coping styles and see the world as less threatening, and thus relax and lower their blood pressure.

In 1939 Alexander published the first results of his efforts. He described a hypertensive patient whom he had seen for over two years of intensive psychoanalytically based psychotherapy. Although Alexander's patient apparently had gained a number of psychodynamic insights from the treatment, after two years of therapy he remained hypertensive. Insight-oriented psychotherapy simply did not appear to be either a cost-effective or a clinically potent way to lower BP. In spite of the disappointing outcome, however, Alexander was able to make a number of observations about what he called the "hypertensive personality," as well as to describe the links between the patient's varying emotional state and baseline BP. When the patient discussed less emotionally provocative material, BP was invariably lower. By contrast, when the patient appeared more agitated or discussed anxiety-provoking material, BP was invariably higher. This finding was so consistent from session to session that it left no doubt in Alexander's mind about the theoretical validity of Cannon's fight/flight response.

Equally intriguing were Alexander's descriptions of the patient's personality—observations subsequently confirmed by a large number of other investigators over the next two decades (Wolf and others, 1955; Graham, Kabler, and Graham, 1962; Weiner, 1979). Alexander traced the patient's personality conflicts and the etiology of hypertension back to struggles in early childhood. Noting among other facts that his patient's father was a severe alcoholic, Alexander hypothesized that the patient had experienced serious dysfunctional communications in his childhood and had come to feel hopeless about expressing himself to others in adulthood. In his early life, the patient's needs to be cared for, soothed, and understood were not adequately met.* Extrapolating from early developmental experiences, Alexander hypothesized that the hypertensive patient's unfulfilled need for support and affection had led to the development of dependent relationships in which the patient repressed hostile or negative feelings for fear of provoking others into anger and rejection. Driven to seek acceptance and support from others, the patient tried to appear friendly although he was actually dominated by excessive but inhibited hostility.

Subsequent clinical confirmations of Alexander's psychodynamic formulations of the hypertensive personality have been frequently criticized for their subjectivity; nevertheless, as Weiner (1979) has noted, so many studies have reported similar findings that one has to be impressed with the concurrent validity of the observations. The general consensus is that, at least for a portion of the hypertensive population, there is a "hypertensive personality" characterized by lifelong but unconscious conflicts about the expression of hostility, aggression, resentment, rage, dependency, ambition, and rebellion. Interpersonal interactions therefore pose a constant threat, since they force these patients to confront their own rage. This, in turn, has the potential to trigger fight/flight responses, including rapid elevations in BP.

The recognition of hypertensive patients' emotional reactivity in interpersonal situations unfortunately also posed serious problems for psychotherapeutic approaches to the treatment of this disease. It gradually became obvious that stressful interviews or stressful psychotherapeutic encounters would force hypertensive patients to respond in a fight-or-flight mode, whereas the therapeutic setting permitted neither fight nor

---

*A psychoanalytic colleague, Herbert S. Gross, interpreted this observation and subsequent findings in our clinic at the University of Maryland Medical School to suggest that hypertensive patients never learn the relaxation response, including lowering BP, early in life and thus become conditioned to a chronic hypertensive state of fight/flight.

flight. The magnitude of this problem was outlined with striking clarity by Wolf and associates (1955) in their text *Life Stress and Essential Hypertension.* In a series of compelling studies—aimed at proving that emotional stress, especially the recall of earlier life traumas, has a major influence on BP and that life stress is a major, if not *the single most important,* cause of essential hypertension—they documented the hemodynamic changes that occur in hypertensive patients during stressful interviews. Specifically, conflict about the open expression of aggressive feelings in stressful interviews put these patients into an extreme state of emotional arousal. The cardiovascular price of this conflict was documented in the truly extraordinary BP increases observed in hypertensive patients during the course of thirty-minute stress interviews (Wolf and Wolff, 1951). In hundreds of patients, major changes in renal flow, glomerular filtration rates, clotting time, peripheral resistance, stroke volume, and epinephrine and norepinephrine levels were recorded during these interviews. Moreover, although reassurance and more relaxed interviews did lead to a transient lowering of BP, the data implied that insight-oriented psychotherapy was not likely to be an effective way to lower BP.

In light of these findings, investigators began to examine the interactive coping styles of hypertensive patients—especially in their interactions with authority figures (Weiner, 1979; Thaler, Weiner, and Reiser, 1957; Graham, Kabler, and Graham, 1960, 1962; Graham, 1962). These investigators observed that hypertensive patients perceive other people as sources of danger and potential derision, and generally as untrustworthy. Because of these perceptions, they try to maintain distance in their social relationships: "Hypertensive subjects were more unreactive physiologically than normotensive ones, because they interacted little with the experimenter. One hypertensive subject who had previously been unresponsive physiologically was persuaded against his will to undergo the laboratory procedure on a second occasion. He equated the second experiment with a threat to his life, his distant style crumbled, and a very brisk, long-lasting blood pressure response occurred. . . . Hypertensive patients have individual styles of relating to physicians and experimenters in the laboratory. They keep their distance from them and avoid close personal involvements. They forgo relationships because they perceive the physician as hostile, dangerous, coercive, or ungiving. If they cannot avoid the relationship, their blood pressure responses are brisker and more prolonged than those of normotensive patients" (Weiner, 1979, pp. 38-39). Unfortunately, these efforts to maintain distance may lead others to detect the hypertensive individual's distance and suspiciousness, frequently provoking the very response he fears most —that is, reciprocal distrust and anger (Weiner, 1979). These findings implied that psychotherapeutic efforts—if they unwittingly intruded on the social-distancing defense mechanisms of hypertensive patients—probably would produce full-blown fight/flight hypertensive reactions.

By the time that antihypertensive drugs began to appear in the early 1950s, several psychodynamic and psychophysiological aspects of hypertensive patients were fairly well established. First of all, there appeared to be a constellation of factors that made psychotherapy a problematic mode of treatment, even though there was virtually unanimous agreement that emotional arousal was a significant component of the disease. There was also widespread agreement that certain psychodynamic defense patterns appeared with regularity in hypertensive patients. Prominent among these were social distancing and repression of rage. Psychotherapeutic attempts to bridge this gap unfortunately appeared to stir either psychodynamic resistance or emotional upheaval, leading to marked increases in BP. Thus, psychotherapy did not appear to be an effective treatment modality. At the same time, certain aspects of the therapeutic relationship—namely, reassurance and support from the therapist, along with instructions to relax—did seem effective in transiently lowering BP.

In an extensive study of the effectiveness of reassurance and support in lowering BP in hypertensive patients, Reiser and his associates (1951) examined ninety-eight hypertensive patients who were given three different levels of therapeutic support. Significant reductions in BP were observed in 22-58 percent of the patients, while 20 percent of the patients had higher

BP at the end of therapy. The most intensive of the therapeutic interactions was described as "superficial insight therapy," thus differentiating it from the more traditional modes of insight-oriented psychotherapy. Over a two-year period, almost half of the population was able to derive some benefit from this inter-action, with success apparently linked to the hypertensive pa-tients' ability to maintain their unconscious defense mecha-nisms and distance in the therapeutic relationship.

In 1956 Moses, Daniels, and Nickerson described ten pa-tients who were seen in intensive psychoanalytically oriented insight therapy. Interestingly, the patients varied in the severity of their disease. The four patients described as "transiently hy-pertensive" became normotensive after six months of therapy. By contrast, the two with the highest BP readings, labeled "ac-celerated hypertension" (200-230/110-130), discontinued treatment. One other severely hypertensive patient reduced his pressure from 220-260/130-150 to 160-190/100-110. The others maintained pressure at borderline hypertensive levels. Those who were most severely hypertensive apparently could not tolerate insight-oriented psychotherapy and so withdrew from the treatment.

The reports by Wolf, Reiser, and Moses and colleagues were to be the last of their kind for several decades, for during that same period there was a rapid expansion of pharmacologi-cal agents to treat hypertension. The effectiveness of drugs and the time-consuming and costly nature of analytically oriented psychotherapy, as well as its questionable effectiveness, led to an abrupt cessation of interest in this dimension of hypertensive management and an accompanying loss of interest in the power-ful links that had been demonstrated between interpersonal interactions and BP. Interest shifted instead back toward inter-nal mechanisms, or physiological factors involved in the regula-tion of BP. Curiously, when subsequent interest in nonpharma-cological approaches would surface again, they would parallel drug approaches insofar as they focused on mechanistic control of BP. That is, both the pharmacological and subsequent non-pharmacological approaches tended to ignore the interpersonal dimensions of BP regulation. As we shall see, this shift in focus

of interest posed serious conceptual and methodological problems for the nonpharmacological approaches; for, in spite of
their focus on techniques, they were essentially interpersonal in
nature. That is, whether the specific approach focused on meditation or relaxation or biofeedback, another person or teacher
was involved to some degree as an inherent part of the therapeutic technique.

Relaxation and Meditation

At virtually the same time that Alexander first published
his studies on hypertension, Jacobson (1939) developed an approach called progressive relaxation. Jacobson's approach was
based on precisely the same theoretical assumptions that Alexander accepted as the basis for his use of psychotherapy to treat
hypertension. Similarly recognizing the implications of Cannon's research, Jacobson set out to develop a relaxation technique that might successfully address the links between emotional arousal, stress, and bodily dysfunction. He was particularly
interested in the skeletal muscular correlates of emotional
arousal, assuming that patients needed to learn how to relax
muscles that were in a spastic state of chronic tension—that is,
chronic fight/flight. Jacobson believed that a person should first
deal with the somatic symptoms of chronic fight/flight and that
such symptomatic relief was a necessary first step in the treatment process. His conceptual framework is important to understand because it influenced many subsequent relaxation techniques. While the empirical foundations of his approach were
similar to Alexander's, his treatment was totally different. In
general, he ignored issues surrounding interpersonal relationships and cardiovascular regulation and focused instead on
techniques of relaxation, assuming that anyone could avail himself of these techniques regardless of the psychodynamic origins
of his conflicts. If these techniques were useful in lowering BP,
presumably they would generalize and thus help individuals deal
with their interpersonal lives.

In 1920 Jacobson published his first observations on
hypertensive patients. He observed that they characteristically

held various skeletal muscles somewhat rigid and overcontrolled
and that their movements were hypertonic. He began to experiment with techniques that would help these patients relax their
muscles through direct training in progressive relaxation. While
the results of his early studies were inconsistent, he did note
that muscle relaxation training could help some patients gradually lower their BP. He documented that the deliberate tensing
of muscle groups would lead to transient elevations in pressure
and that the more vigorous the tensing, the greater the BP increases. His studies showing a lowering of baseline BP, however,
were less convincing because of differences in sample size and
variations in treatment modes, duration of treatment, and duration of follow-up studies. They were important, however, in
suggesting that muscle relaxation is an indirect way to regulate
BP. The technique was labeled "progressive" to suggest that—
with practice and concentrated, focused relaxation on ever
more specific skeletal muscle groups—individuals would become
progressively more adept at relaxing.

Jacobson's research formed the basis for a variety of relaxation techniques that differ somewhat in orientation. Some
emphasize cognitive dimensions of relaxation (meditation),
while others focus on physiological aspects of relaxation, especially deep breathing and muscle relaxation. In a comprehensive
review of various behavioral methods for the treatment of hypertension, Shapiro and his associates (1977) list seven types of
relaxation. Among those techniques used to lower BP, they cite
the following methods:

1. Progressive relaxation as outlined by Jacobson.
2. Autogenic training, first described by Luthe (1969). This
    technique involves a form of self-hypnosis or autosugges-
    tion in which a person (usually with the aid of an instructor-
    therapist) gives himself suggestions and repeats these sug-
    gestions (for example, "My legs feel warm and relaxed")
    over and over again.
3. Hypnotic relaxation induced by a hypnotherapist.
4. Zen meditation, involving quiet concentration and special

focus on one's respiration, coupled with various exercises that elicit the relaxation response.

5.   Hatha yoga, which is similar to Zen in its emphasis on breathing and meditation but adds an additional focus on the effects of various bodily posture states.

6.   Transcendental meditation (TM), which involves a cognitive focus. In this relaxation technique, an individual sits quietly in a comfortable position; closes his eyes; and softly repeats a specific "Mantra," usually a Sanskrit word or sound, while he slowly exhales his breath.

7.   The "relaxation response" standardized by Benson and his co-workers at Harvard. This technique is based on the principles of transcendental meditation but was tailored to suit Western cultures (Benson and Wallace, 1972).

With the exception of Benson's relaxation response, none of these relaxation techniques was originally designed specifically to lower BP. Yet each was found to lower overall emotional arousal and thus have nonspecific benefits, including the lowering of BP. Table 1 lists a variety of published relaxation studies, as well as the magnitude of pressure reductions reported in these studies. It is difficult to interpret the results of these studies because they varied markedly in patient samples, pretreatment baseline pressures, medications, and magnitude of effects; nevertheless, the trends toward lower BP are similar in virtually every study.

While all these studies report some statistically significant lowering of BP, the reductions in BP vary greatly, from 17 to 4 mm Hg systolic and from 16 to 0 mm Hg diastolic. The crucial test in reduction of blood pressure is in the number of subjects who were able to lower their BPs to a clinically safe level (140/90). Most studies report only mean reductions in group blood pressures. It is therefore difficult to determine how many individual patients attained the therapeutic goal of 140/90. Jacobson (1939) reports individual data, and one of his three patients lowered BP from 172/82 to 165/68. Bali (1979), who also discusses subjects as individuals, reports that only two out of

Table 1. Blood Pressure Reductions in Relaxation Studies.

Researcher	N	Technique	Reduction: Systolic/Diastolic	Follow-Up
Jacobson (1939)	3	Progressive relaxation	17/9	None
Taylor and others (1977)	11	Progressive relaxation	14/5	6 mo.
Bali (1979)	17	Progressive relaxation	12/9	12 mo.
Stone and DeLeo (1976)	19	Zen meditation	9/8	None
Datey and others (1969)	10[a]	Hatha yoga	15 (MAP)[d]	None
	15[b]		10 (MAP)	
	22[c]		2 (MAP)	
Benson and others (1974a)	14	Transcendental meditation	11/5	None
Benson and others (1974b)	22	Transcendental meditation	6/4	None
Blackwell and others (1976)	7	Transcendental meditation	4/.2	6 mo.
Pollack and others (1977)	20	Transcendental meditation	9/0	6 mo.
Crowther (1983)	12	Imagery	13/12	6 mo.
	12	Stress management	13/16	6 mo.
Southam and others (1982)	10	Relaxation	14/12	15 mo.

[a]Patients who received no medication.

[b]Patients whose medication did not control their blood pressure.

[c]Patients whose medication did control their blood pressure.

[d]MAP = mean arterial pressure.

seventeen subjects had clinically significant reductions (142/90 to 122/76 and 144/97 to 122/80). Crowther (1983) states that eighteen of the twenty-four in the combined groups (stress management and mental imagery) obtained normal BPs and that the other six had marked reductions in medication.

Another crucial question is the effectiveness of the treatment result upon follow-up. Recent work has shown that relaxation training can result in twenty-four-hour reductions in BP after treatment (Agras, 1983; Agras and others, 1980) and in decreases at the work site (Southam and others, 1982). There are also a few studies that report longer follow-up: Blackwell and associates (1976), Crowther (1983), and Taylor and associates (1977) did six-month follow-up evaluations. Blackwell found that two out of five subjects sustained their decreases. Crowther reports sustained reductions at six months, Bali at twelve months, and Agras, Southam, and Taylor at fifteen months. By contrast, Pollack and associates (1977) report that the benefits of relaxation training were not maintained at a six-month follow-up. Thus, the relaxation studies show inconsistent and mixed results from their training protocols.

The most impressive and consistent of the therapeutic benefits of a mixed relaxation approach have been reported by Patel and her co-workers. Her approach involves a combination of meditation, relaxation, biofeedback, and, in one study, a technique that she labels stress management (Patel, Marmot, and Terry, 1981). The magnitude of the decreases in BP range from 26 to 14 mm Hg for systolic pressure and 16 to 7 mm Hg for diastolic BP. In addition, unlike most other reports, Patel conducted follow-up studies nine months after therapy and found that the therapeutic benefits were maintained. A summary of the results from her studies can be seen in Table 2. Patel reports that these results were maintained on follow-up visits.

While it is not clear why Patel's approach produced consistently greater results than those reported by other investigators using relaxation methods, a nonspecific factor seems to distinguish her approach. She consistently emphasizes the importance of being a warm and supportive therapist during the training

Table 2. BP Reductions in Relaxation Studies Reported by Patel.

	N	Technique	BP Reduction (mm Hg)	Follow-Up
Patel (1973)	20	Relaxation, meditation, and feedback	26/16	None
Patel (1975a)	20	Relaxation, meditation, and feedback	20/14	9 mo.
	20	Control	+.5/+2.1	
Patel and North (1975)	17	Relaxation, meditation, and feedback	27/16	3 mo.
	17	Control	9/4	
Patel and Datey (1976)	27	Relaxation and feedback	17/13	6 mo.
	20	Control	.5/.1	
Patel, Marmot, and Terry (1981)	99	Relaxation, feedback, and stress management	14/7	8 mo.
	93	Control	4/1.4	

exercises; and she also emphasizes a more common component, the importance of deep breathing during relaxation. However, in light of the powerful nonspecific effects of variables such as status differences on blood pressure (Long and others, 1982), embedded nonspecific factors in Patel's approach need to be more carefully considered.

BP reductions in relaxation studies are often difficult to interpret because the studies fail to distinguish between BP reductions that are statistically significant and those that are clinically significant. Again, Patel's studies are an exception in this regard. In two of her studies (Patel, 1973; Patel and Datey, 1976), issues surrounding the clinical effectiveness of her treatment are specifically addressed. Combining the patients from these two studies ($N = 47$), one finds that 25 percent of her patients (thirteen of forty-seven) stopped all medications and could maintain their BP within normotensive ranges during follow-up visits. Eight additional patients reduced the amount of medications by 33-67 percent while still maintaining normal pressures. Ten did not alter their medicines but were able to maintain normotensive BP levels, while six had variable changes in medicines but could not lower either systolic below 140 or diastolic BP below 90. Finally, ten patients were considered treatment failures because there was no change in medications, and they could not lower their BP below 160/90.

Biofeedback

Of all the nonpharmacological treatment approaches, probably none has generated more intense scientific and clinical interest than an approach popularly known as biofeedback. This approach suggests that if a patient is given "feedback" (via tones, lights, or digitalized information) about a bodily function such as BP, the individual can utilize this information to gain control of that function. For example, if a person's BP is too high, then feedback about this fact should allow the patient to learn ways to lower it to more normal levels.

While the term has been used in a variety of contexts and has taken on a number of different meanings, biofeedback as a

theoretical construct owes its origins to the research of Neal
Miller. As used by Miller and his associates (Miller, 1969; Miller
and Dworkin, 1977; DiCara and Miller, 1978) and by Shapiro
and his associates (1977), biofeedback denotes a very specific
methodological approach—namely, operant conditioning, which
is applied to the control of various visceral systems. As used in a
clinical context, however, the term "biofeedback" is used to describe different methodological approaches that often have little
in common. This imprecise use of the term has in turn made it
very difficult to compare the studies purporting to use this
methodological approach to treat hypertension.

From a conceptual point of view, the term "biofeedback" first arose when Miller presented empirical evidence suggesting that certain traditional assumptions about learning theory were inaccurate. Historically, psychologists had posited two
types of conditioning or learning: one called classical or Pavlovian conditioning; the other, instrumental, operant, or Skinnerian conditioning. Psychologists had traditionally believed that
Pavlovian conditioning, in which a tone was paired with a reinforcement, primarily influenced the autonomic visceral nervous
system. The reinforcement was presented to the animal no matter how it responded during the conditional signal. In technical
terms this was called "noncontingent reinforcement," since the
reinforcement was not contingent (dependent) on the nature of
the animal's response. While such responses included the skeletal muscular system of animals, generally the focus was on the
autonomic conditional reactions that occurred during the conditional signal. Operant or Skinnerian conditioning, by contrast,
focused almost exclusively on the somatic or skeletal responses
of an animal. An animal first had to emit a response, which was
then reinforced by food or avoidance of shock; and by the suc-
cessive pairing of responses with reinforcements, the behavior of
the animal was "shaped." The reinforcement was contingent—
that is, dependent on the animal's response—and so the focus
was quite naturally on those aspects of the nervous system response that were under an animal's voluntary control.

Thus, Pavlovian conditioning was supposed to influence
the autonomic or involuntary nervous system, whereas Skinner-

ian conditioning was supposed to influence the voluntary or skeletal muscular system. Miller challenged this distinction by asserting that operant conditioning techniques could be used to control the autonomic nervous system. That is, an animal's autonomic nervous system could be "contingently reinforced" and the behavior systems heretofore considered involuntary brought under voluntary control. An animal's heart rate, for example, could be brought under contingent control in precisely the same way that an animal used his skeletal muscles to press a bar "contingently" to get a food reward. In essence, Miller was asserting that the historically accepted differences between the voluntary and involuntary nervous systems needed to be redefined and that the visceral, or involuntary, nervous system could be brought under voluntary control.

In a series of remarkable experiments (most of which could not be replicated and were found to have serious methodological flaws), Miller (1969) ostensibly demonstrated that specific autonomic nervous system functions—such as heart rate, blood flow, blood pressure, salivation, and gastrointestinal motility—could be shaped to perform in roughly the same way that an animal had been trained to press a key to obtain food. That is, by "contingently rewarding" an animal whenever it increased its heart rate—for example, by giving a curarized animal a burst of electrical stimulation in a pleasure center of its brain—one could teach the animal to increase its heart rate. Conversely, other animals could be taught to slow their heart rates in precisely the same way. When they were "rewarded" for slowing their heart rate, it could slow down even to the point of cardiac arrest.

Although these studies and the conceptual framework that guided them were subsequently shown to be fraught with problems (not the least of which was that the phrase "voluntary control of the involuntary nervous system" is a contradiction in terms), they stimulated clinicians to begin exploring "biofeedback" for the treatment of a variety of psychosomatic disorders (Lynch, 1973). Virtually overnight there was an explosion of research interest, and the techniques were applied to a broad array of clinical problems. Within a few years, a number of studies purporting to use biofeedback (that is, contingent feedback) to control hypertension began to appear. Although these studies had ostensibly used the same methodological approach—that is, feedback of blood pressure—they varied significantly on a number of crucial methodological issues as well as on outcome. As was true of earlier relaxation reports, these biofeedback studies varied in populations examined, follow-up, medications, and other features. They also generally reported some lowering of BP. In most of the "pure" biofeedback studies, however, its effectiveness in lowering BP had to be considered marginal at best.

Of all the methodological problems, perhaps none was more crucial than the blurring of interpersonal issues with biofeedback techniques. Lynch and associates (1982b) examined these biofeedback studies, along with a variety of other nonpharmacological treatment approaches for hypertension, and found that most studies had seriously underestimated the importance of interpersonal issues in their treatment protocols. As Table 3 indicates, simple objective factors—such as time spent, the number of sessions, the technique employed, or the inclusion of home practice—fail to explain a large part of the variance in the results. An examination of certain interpersonal issues, however, reveals another hidden influence:

> One way of examining these influences is to categorize studies as clinical or experimental studies and evaluate the reductions in BP. In this regard, experimental studies were assumed to place the subject alone during training, to refer to participants as subjects, to have a fixed script or protocol, and to present the study to participants as experimental and episodic in nature, while therapeutic studies were assumed to embody the opposite characteristics. If these studies are divided on the basis of their possessing two or more characteristics, twenty-five of the total of thirty-five studies could be classified. Eleven were judged therapeutic in orientation, and fourteen were judged experimental. . . . The average decreases [in systolic and diastolic BP] for studies judged experimental were 8/5 mm Hg, while for those studies judged therapeutic the reductions were 16/10, or twice the re-

duction. One additional factor also influences this apparent relationship. Some of the studies carried out in the therapeutic context used participants with somewhat higher initial BP (mean therapeutic = 156/99; mean experimental = 148/96). An analysis of the relationship between initial pressure and subsequent reductions after treatment reveals a significant correlation ($r = .65, p < .01$) for systolic pressure, although for diastolic pressure the correlation is insignificant ($r = .02$). Such a relationship has been mentioned previously (Jacob, Kraemer, and Agras, 1977), but more attention needs to be given to this factor in future studies. An explanation for the systolic-diastolic difference may rest in a relative emphasis on systolic pressure reductions in these studies. For example, five studies have focused on systolic pressure alone, while only one has limited measurement to diastolic pressure [Lynch and others, 1982b, p. 146].

While some recent biofeedback studies have failed to control adequately for the influence of the therapist in the treatment program, other investigators have made systematic efforts to contrast the effectiveness of biofeedback with that of other approaches. For example, Frankel and associates (1978) compared biofeedback and relaxation with a sham treatment and control group. They did not observe differences in any of the groups. Only one out of twenty-two patients significantly lowered BP (from 145/95 to 127/85) and maintained that decrease at an eighteen-month follow-up visit.

In 1975 Shoemaker and Tasto described one of the first controlled comparison studies of relaxation versus biofeedback. They reported that only relaxation decreased both systolic and diastolic BP significantly (7/8) from pretreatment to posttreatment; biofeedback alone was less effective in lowering diastolic BP.

Walsh, Dale, and Anderson (1977) again compared relaxation and biofeedback and then combined them as a second phase of treatment. Neither individual treatment was found to be significantly more effective, and combined feedback and relaxation led to no greater decreases. All three treatment modali-

Table 3. Behavioral Hypertension Studies and Their Characteristics.

Study	Date	No. of Subjects	No. of Sessions	Session Length (minutes)	Home Practice	Person Present	Interaction	Participant	Goal	Blood Pressure	
										Initial	Decrease
Jacobson	1939	3	5	90	?	Yes	?	Patient	?	172/94	17/9
Datey and others	1969	10	15	30	Yes	Yes	Script	Patient	?	185/109	37/23
Benson and others	1971	7	8-34	60	No	?	Ad lib	Subject	Study	165/X[a]	16/X
Deabler, Fidel, Dillenkoffer	1973	6	8	35	Yes	Yes	Script	?	Treat	163/96	28/16
Elder and others	1973	6	8	30	No	Yes	Script	Patient	?	154/104	+2/6
	1973	6	8	30	No	Yes	?	Patient	?	151/108	23/10
Patel	1973	20	36	30	Yes	?	?	Patient	?	160/102	26/16
Benson and others	1974b	22	11	20	Yes	No	Script	Subject	Study	147/95	6/4
Brady, Luborsky, Kron	1974	4	14-22	30	Yes	?	Script	Subject	Study	X/105	X/3
Redmond and others	1974	6	5	30	Yes	?	?	Subject	Study	141/101	7/2
Blanchard, Young, Haynes	1975	4	2	40	No	No	?	Subject	Study	154/X	17/X
Elder and Eustis	1975	22	10	60	No	No	?	Subject	Study	147/85	8/4
Goldman and others	1975	7	9	120	Yes	?	?	Subject	Study	167/109	8/15
Kristt and Engel	1975	5	3	20	Yes	No	Ad lib	Patient	?	152/X	18/X
Patel	1975a	20	39	30	Yes	?	?	Patient	?	159/100	20/14
Patel	1975b	16	12	30	Yes	?	?	Patient	?	156/98	12/11
Patel and North	1975	17	12	60	Yes	?	?	Patient	Treat	168/100	27/16
Shapiro and others	1975	6	5	30	No	Yes	?	Patient	Study	142/101	4/6
Shoemaker and Tasto	1975	5	6	80	No	Yes	Script	Subject	Study	143/92	7/8
Patel and Datey	1976	27	27	30	Yes	?	?	Patient	?	158/99	17/13
Stone and DeLeo	1976	14	10-14	5-20	Yes	?	?	Patient	?	146/90	9/8
Kleinman and others	1977	8	9	120	Yes	?	?	Subject	?	149/93	6/8
Pollack and others	1977	20	16	20	Yes	?	?	Patient	?	155/96	9/0

Taylor and others	1977	11	5	30	Yes	Yes	Ad lib	Patient	?	150/96	14/5
	1977	10	5	30	No	Yes	Ad lib	Patient	?	141/92	3/2
Friedman and Taub	1977	13	6	20	No	?	?	Subject	Study	147/96	8/6
		10	6	20	Yes	?	?	Subject	Study	140/92	1/3
Beiman, Graham, Ciminero	1978	2	7-8	50	Yes	?	?	Patient	?	143/93	17/9
Christoph and others	1978	18	1	48	No	No	Script	Subject	?	139/94	1/1
Frankel and others	1978	7	20	45	Yes	No	?	Subject	Study	150/96	4/3
Patel and others	1978	4	20	30	No	?	?	Patient	?	149/98	2/2
Surwit, Shapiro, Good	1978	24	8	60	Yes	No	Script	Subject	Study	141/X	+3/X
Blanchard and others	1979	28	12	40	Yes	No	Script	Patient	Study	146/95	8/1
Bertilson, Bartz, Zimmerman	1979	8	14-22	12	No	Yes	Script	Subject	?	139/82	21/X
Green, Green, Norris	1979	12	28	45	Yes	?	?	Patient	Treat	142/93	7/7

[a]X = Not given in article.

Source: Adapted from Lynch and others (1982b).

ties, however, were effective in lowering BP significantly, and a one-year follow-up indicated that the BP decreases were maintained.

In an effort to evaluate the effectiveness of biofeedback in the treatment of borderline essential hypertension, Blanchard and his colleagues (1979) compared direct BP feedback with frontalis EMG feedback and self-instructed relaxation. Patients were also followed up for four months after treatment, and the generalization of the effectiveness of treatment was assessed by reports of BP recorded in the physician's office. None of the treatments led to a significant reduction in diastolic BP, but systolic BP fell 8.1 mm Hg for patients receiving BP feedback and 9.5 mm Hg for relaxation patients. In the physician's office, only patients who had received relaxation training showed a significant drop in BP.

Surwit, Shapiro, and Good (1978) evaluated the relative effectiveness of BP biofeedback, frontalis muscle feedback, and meditation (Benson's relaxation response) in the treatment of borderline hypertension. Patients were examined for two baseline sessions, eight training sessions, and a six-week follow-up. Although all groups showed modest reductions in BP from pretreatment levels, there were no significant differences between the treatment groups. At one-year follow-up, BP did not differ from pretreatment levels.

Luborsky and associates (1982) compared the relative effectiveness (for hypertensive patients) of antihypertensive medicines, relaxation training, biofeedback, and mild exercise. Each group was given six weeks of treatment. Those given medications achieved the largest decreases in BP. The biofeedback and relaxation and mild exercise groups all lowered pressure somewhat but did not significantly differ from each other.

Engel, Glasglow, and Gaarder (1983) have recently reported the results of a highly complex study of ninety mild hypertensive patients. They compared relaxation (RR), biofeedback (FF), biofeedback followed by relaxation (FR), and relaxation followed by biofeedback (RF). They also used extensive home monitoring of BP. They observed that these various treatment modalities had a variable effect on BP. FR proved to be most effective, with reductions of 13.8/10.2; RF ranked second in effectiveness (8.0/5.6); then RR (6.2/7.0); and finally FF (4.7/6.2). These decreases were sustained at six-month follow-up visits. Forty-four patients were taking medicines (diuretics); of these, thirteen (ten in the FR group and three in the RF group) were able to discontinue medications because of a sustained lowering of diastolic pressure below 90 mm Hg. These results led the investigators to propose a stepped-care (nonpharmacological) approach, which included self-monitoring of BP, followed by feedback, followed by relaxation.

To date, feedback alone has not proved effective in lowering BP in hypertensives. The combination approach (feedback with relaxation) seems to be somewhat more effective.

From all the previous literature on nonpharmacological aspects of BP regulation, several conclusions can be drawn:

1. Interpersonal interactions, particularly those that are emotionally stressful, can elicit major increases in BP.
2. Therapeutic interactions that emphasize reassurance and emotional support can lead to rapid, transient reductions in BP.
3. A variety of nonpharmacological methods—including relaxation, meditation, and biofeedback—all report some degree of success in lowering BP in hypertensive patients.
4. While relaxation, biofeedback, and meditation emphasize different procedural techniques, they all involve interpersonal interactions, the effects of which have not been carefully assessed in the observed therapeutic outcomes.
5. The very measurement of BP itself is inherently interpersonal—a fact that may have significantly influenced the findings of both pharmacological and nonpharmacological studies.
6. Talking has a potent influence on the cardiovascular system and can lead to immediate increases in BP.
7. All the nonpharmacological approaches, other than psychotherapy, structurally build *silence* into their treatment protocols, a fact that might have accounted for the BP reductions observed quite apart from any specific approach that was employed.
8. Issues surrounding interpersonal relationships and the over-

all regulation of BP have to be carefully assessed regardless of which nonpharmacological treatment one is considering.

Effects of Human Communication and Social Distancing on Blood Pressure

While a number of interpersonal factors appear to play a major role in the overall regulation of blood pressure, certain of these factors appear to be paradoxically at odds with each other. For example, evidence indicates that human loneliness is a significant contributor to cardiovascular disease and cardiovascular mortality (Lynch, 1979). Mortality statistics reveal that single, widowed, and divorced individuals have significantly higher death rates from coronary heart disease, hypertension, and other cardiovascular disease (Lynch, 1979). On the other hand, the data reviewed earlier indicate that stressful social encounters can cause significant elevations in the BP of hypertensive patients. Perhaps the success of treatment approaches such as meditation, relaxation, and biofeedback stems from the fact that these approaches are solitary in character and involve treatment protocols in which patients usually remain quiet. However, these treatments do not address the fundamental social isolation and social-distancing problems that also seem to play a role in the "dis-ease" of many hypertensive patients. Like everyone else, hypertensive patients must live in a social world. Mortality statistics suggest that hypertensive individuals would face an increased risk of cardiovascular disease if they withdrew from social contact on a continual basis. At the same time, studies indicate that hypertensive individuals can experience very real stress, accompanied by marked surges in BP, when they try to interact with other people. Thus, these patients appear to be trapped no matter which course they choose.

The paradox of hypertensive dialogue was of central concern to us when we began to monitor the effects of interpersonal interactions on BP with a computerized BP machine.* Be-

*We are grateful to David A. Paskewitz of Digital Psychophysiological Systems, Inc., Baltimore, for helping to develop the Blood Pressure Profile System used in our studies.

cause the computerized machine automatically inflates the cuff and records blood pressure and heart rate every minute, and displays the information digitally, we were able to observe that every time our hypertensive patients spoke, their BP rose, and as soon as we (as therapists) began to talk, their BP fell to pretalking levels (Lynch and others, 1982a). The rise in BP seemed to be an additive phenomenon, one that included the act of talking as well as the emotional content of the dialogue. The magnitude and rapidity of the BP changes were truly remarkable. At times the patients' BP rose almost 50 percent above baseline levels within thirty seconds after they began talking, and it fell just as quickly when they were quiet once again.

At first we assumed that this response could be attributed to a peculiar combination of the disease of hypertension and the stressful nature of our clinical interviews. That interpretation was based primarily on the earlier conclusions of Alexander (1939) and Wolf and Wolff (1951). Thus, we thought it unlikely that comparable BP increases would occur outside the therapeutic milieu or in normotensive individuals. But our assumption proved to be incorrect: For virtually all ages, both sexes, and all races, we found that blood pressure and heart rate increased anywhere from 10 to 50 percent as soon as people began to speak. Beyond the ubiquity of the response, we also observed a strong positive correlation between baseline pressure and the magnitude of the elevations during talking (Lynch and others, 1981). The higher a person's resting BP, the more it tended to rise when he began to speak. Hypertensive individuals exhibited highly significant elevations in BP even though most of them were taking conventional antihypertensive medications (Lynch and others, 1981; Malinow and others, 1982).

While these observations raised a number of questions about hypertension, they also suggested that the marked increases in BP observed in earlier studies might have been caused not merely by the emotional stress of the interview but by the simple act of speaking. In virtually all earlier studies, the focus had been on the affective content of the communication, rather than on the act of communicating; similarly, little attention had been paid to who was speaking (the patient or the therapist) just before the measurement of BP.

After completing a variety of studies testing for the ubiquity of the blood pressure/talking response, we began to explore various factors that influenced the magnitude of increases in BP while talking. One of the more crucial was the rate of speech. Fast talking was followed by significantly higher elevations in BP than normal or slow rates of speech (Friedmann and others, 1982). Breathing patterns during speech also influenced the magnitude of the rise; hypertensive patients in particular appeared to speak in a breathless pattern (Lynch and others, 1982b).

The fact that rapid speech was linked to marked elevations in BP helped us link our observations in hypertensive patients to the coronary-prone (Type A) behavior pattern described by Friedman and Rosenman (Rosenman and others, 1964). (This behavior pattern is discussed in detail in Chapter Four.) They had previously found that Type A personalities have significantly higher cardiac morbidity and mortality rates than Type B personalities do. Prominent among the behavioral traits of Type A personalities are their speech patterns; they tend to speak rapidly and with a great deal of emphasis. Friedman and Rosenman assumed that these rapid and emphatic speech patterns constitute a personality trait linked to the Type A character; our data, however, suggested that such speech patterns have a more direct influence on the cardiovascular system (Friedmann and others, 1982).

The striking relationship between talking and rapid elevations in BP also suggested that communication and communicative styles have a powerful influence on the cardiovascular system and that the disorder of hypertension might be the result of, or seriously exacerbated by, dysfunctions in communication. It appeared as if some hypertensive patients might literally have talked their way into this disorder. This hypothesis naturally led us to wonder whether they could be taught communicative styles that would allow them to talk their way out of this problem.

Transactional Psychophysiology:
A Brief Description of a New Approach

The observations of the direct relationship between speaking and BP, as well as the hypotheses that these observations helped generate, gradually led to the development of a new approach to the treatment of hypertension. The approach not only emphasized the minute-to-minute digital feedback of blood pressure and heart rate but also linked these changes to shifts in dialogue within the context of human verbal interactions. It became obvious that an approach similar to, yet fundamentally different from, that originally employed by Alexander might help bridge the gap between the vascular consequences of loneliness and the hypertensive patient's needs for social distancing. Since the magnitude of BP increases during speech was significantly correlated with baseline BP (Lynch and others, 1981), it appeared likely that efforts aimed at lowering baseline BP would have the corresponding effect of lowering the magnitude of BP rises when hypertensive individuals talked. In addition, the computerized feedback of BP could be used by the patient and the therapist to titrate the magnitude of pressure rises that could be tolerated before the patient should pause and be instructed to relax and be quiet. The type of approach used by Alexander, in which a patient was monitored only at the beginning and the end of therapy, would not be sensitive to the marked shifts in blood pressure when the patient talked. It also became clear that hypertensive patients with very high pressures would not be able to tolerate insight-oriented psychotherapy, since the physiological concomitants of their ongoing dialogue could be lethal. Since a number of relaxation, meditation, and biofeedback approaches rely on deep breathing and relaxation, it seemed appropriate to incorporate these techniques into periods of quiet during the therapeutic dialogue.

Beyond the technical orientation of titrating human dialogue, it occurred to us that BP rises while speaking could be looked at as a hidden bodily communication, a form of internal blushing, which therapists could use as a psychophysiological signal to alter ongoing dialogue. We also began to recognize that the patient and the therapist share a fundamental problem: Neither can afford to ignore important vascular consequences of their ongoing dialogue. Consequently, the therapeutic approach that we developed—an approach called "transactional psychophysiology" (or TP therapy)—was based on the fundamental idea that every bodily response in human dialogue is a communicative transaction that must be attended to and understood. Al-though a person's cardiovascular responses can be psychophysi-ological in nature, like blushing, they can also be viewed as vas-cular responses that are essentially interpersonal. This notion of blood pressure elevations as a form of hidden internal blushing helped crystallize a way to make therapeutic use of the hyper-tensive patient's needs to maintain social distance. By devising computerized feedback mechanisms that allowed us to titrate the magnitude of pressure rises during speech, we were in fact both detecting and respecting the social-distancing defense me-chanisms of patients. Attempts to break through such defenses would only cause a patient's BP to rise even higher—up to dan-gerously high and possibly physiologically intolerable levels—so that further dialogue would become virtually impossible.

The primary goal of TP therapy therefore centers on low-ering the cardiovascular component of the fight/flight response in hypertensive dialogue. Although patients cannot directly con-trol BP elevations during stressful communications, they can be made aware of such reactions and taught not to ignore them when they talk. They can also be taught to slow their rate of speech, breathe more deeply, relax their muscles, and, if neces-sary, withdraw periodically for brief periods of quiet relaxation. All these maneuvers should help patients lower their blood pres-sure transiently.

The overall goal of lowering the cardiovascular compo-nent of the fight/flight response in hypertensive dialogue is ac-complished through a series of steps. Though each of these steps involves a number of theoretical constructs that space limita-tions preclude us from discussing here, perhaps a brief outline of our general approach will provide enough detail to give some sense of our overall approach.

The first step in this treatment is an intake interview done by a nurse who is a master's-prepared clinical specialist. A nurse was chosen, and the general medical orientation of the therapy emphasized, in order to support the hypertensive de-fense mechanisms. That is, these patients are generally quite re-sistant to psychological interpretation of their vascular prob-lems. Thus, the more the therapeutic approach resembles the traditional medical model, the more willing hypertensive patients appear to be to accept treatment. In the hour-long interview, the patient's medical history is obtained—including onset, duration, and precipitating, aggravating, and alleviating factors of the disease. Also included are questions about associated symptoms and relevant medical problems—such as the presence of diabetes, heart failure, depressed kidney function, or eye damage; the major risk factors of hypertension and cardiovascular disease—that is, positive family history of hypertension, obesity, increased blood sugar, cholesterol, lipids, and cigarette smoking; all medicines currently taken; and previous hospitalization, surgeries, and medications. The patient's social, psychological, family, and occupational history also is obtained by the nurse. The patient is then evaluated with a battery of computerized psychological and psychophysiological tests, including the Minnesota Multiphasic Personality Inventory, the Life Change Index, and the Cornell Medical Index. Patients whose completed medical workup and psychological profile suggest that they have the capacity to undergo this treatment (those with severe elevations on the Psychotic scale of the MMPI are not accepted for TP therapy) are then admitted for treatment.

In the first phase of TP therapy, the patient is shown various maneuvers that can be used to regulate the cardiovascular system. As an initial step, he is taught to observe changes in his own blood pressure as he engages the therapist in dialogue. This process introduces the patient to the notion that major BP changes frequently occur in the body and that human dialogue can have a significant impact on BP. The idea is then gradually introduced that major changes in BP reflect previously undetected changes in emotional arousal. The patient is taught that he must recognize his own feelings so that he can begin to differentiate hypertensive from relaxing dialogue and pleasant from unpleasant social interactions.

After these initial ideas have been taught, the patient is then introduced to the idea of dysfunctional dialogue. While this dysfunction has various components, one of the more important attributes is the discrepancy between one's internal vascular system and his external demeanor. Many hypertensive pa-

tients appear quite peaceful when their BP surges out of control, a fact that would confuse anyone who attempts to communicate with these patients without computer feedback. Since
these dysfunctional communications are an essential part of
hypertension, it is important that those individuals centrally
linked to the patient's communicative life be involved in the
therapeutic process. Thus, TP therapy necessarily involves
teaching the spouse to understand and decode the patient's con-
fusing vascular communications. Both the hypertensive individual and the spouse are exposed to each other's physiological
changes when they speak to each other. In this way the spouse
and the hypertensive learn some of the mechanical and behavioral cues that accompany previously undetected surges in
blood pressure. Computer feedback permits the patient and the
spouse to see the minute-to-minute changes in their pressures
and heart rates as they communicate. They learn that BP is not
a static number but an ever-changing bodily process that is influenced by a variety of bodily mechanisms that they can
control. Both the patient and the spouse are then shown various
mechanisms that cause pressure elevations and various maneuvers
(such as deep breathing) that can be used to lower blood pressure when they communicate.

As part of the overall therapeutic approach, patients are
also instructed to record BP at home both before and after five
minutes of deep breathing. In addition, they are instructed to
identify how they feel just before they take their own pressures.
This instruction is given in order to reinforce continuously the
idea that human feelings are linked to changes in human BP.

As patients begin to observe themselves and their BP,
they learn to link changes in BP with changes in their everyday
lives. They also watch their mates communicate and see the concomitant changes in their pressures and heart rates. Thus, the
initial step in TP therapy includes observation of self and "significant others" and linking the changes in BP to the social
world in which the patient lives.

During this initial phase of TP therapy, emphasis is placed
on supporting the patient while giving as much didactic information about links between human communication and blood

pressure as the patient can absorb. No efforts are made during this phase to "invade" the patient therapeutically or to provide the patient with dynamic insights about hidden psychological or interpersonal conflicts. This process is entered into only after the patient has some sense of mastery over his BP and the capacity to feel changes in BP when he is emotionally upset.

The computerized displays of blood pressure and heart rate graphically emphasize that specific circumstances, people, and situations cause blood pressure to rise. As the individual sees his blood pressure and heart rate react, he begins to explore the meaning of these changes with his therapist and spouse. Thus, he gradually proceeds to Phase II, or what would be recognized as more conventional psychodynamically oriented psychotherapy, in which these changes can be linked specifically to interactions between the patient, spouse, and therapist. The crucial difference between conventional therapy and TP therapy during this phase is that emphasis remains focused on BP. That is, whenever the patient's BP begins to rise into hypertensive ranges, ongoing conversations are interrupted, and the patient is instructed to breathe deeply and relax. In TP therapy blood pressure is viewed as a dynamic response as well as a dynamic communication that must be attended to as carefully as a patient's verbal communications.

By using blood pressure as a barometric indicator of potential hidden emotional storms, the therapist can titrate the dynamic course of therapy. In addition, both the patient and his mate begin to learn that their hidden vascular communications are as important to listen to and decode as their ongoing verbal dialogue. The therapist also emphasizes that continuing to engage in a dialogue with a person whose blood pressure is rising higher and higher is to participate unwittingly in a dialogue that at best is counterproductive and at worst is potentially murderous.

The last phase in therapy involves teaching the patient and his spouse that, since blood pressure and heart rate changes are an inextricable component of all human dialogue, the process must be attended to throughout life. The hypertensive patient is taught that his BP will always tend to rise while he is discussing emotional and difficult interpersonal issues because he has a genetically determined predisposition to respond to anxiety by altering blood pressure. Thus, the patient learns that he will respond physiologically in a way that might be similar to his parents' hypertensive responsiveness to certain interpersonal situations.

Patients usually learn to lower BP after about twelve to twenty sessions, generally in a six-month period. As is true in psychodynamic therapy, a longer period of time is required before the patient is able to handle deeper dynamic issues without becoming acutely hypertensive. Decisions about probing into deeper dynamic conflicts are usually negotiated during the therapy itself. Certain patients either cannot tolerate such probing or choose to focus specifically on mechanisms controlling BP.

Table 4 describes the first eighteen hypertensive patients (sequentially listed) treated in our clinic. The results to date have been highly encouraging. Many of these patients are still involved in therapy, and, as shown in the table, they vary in age, medication history, and cardiovascular pathology. Yet the majority have been able to lower blood pressure and reduce or stop all medications. The longest follow-up to date has been six years. This patient had an average BP of 162/104 when he began therapy in 1977 and a final pressure of 147/81. In addition, he withdrew from medicines. He had been sent to our clinic by a neurologist because of several transient ischemic attacks. In addition, he had previously had a myocardial infarction. Recent follow-up visits (January 1984) revealed his pressure to be averaging 128/82.

Systematic empirical evaluation of this therapeutic approach is currently in progress, and firm conclusions regarding its efficacy cannot as yet be reached. We are, nonetheless, as clinicians remarkably impressed with the results that have emerged, and we feel that transactional psychophysiology offers the hope of integrating a wealth of psychodynamic insights, developed over decades, with recent technological advances, as well as with findings emerging from behavioral medicine.

Table 4. Blood Pressure Data on the First Eighteen Patients Undergoing Transactional Psychophysiology (TF) Therapy.

COMPLETED SUCCESSFUL

Patient No.	1	2	3	4	5	6
Age	50	37	58	33	46	22
Race/Sex/Mar. Status	W/M/M	W/M/M	W/M/M	W/M/M	W/F/D	W/M/M
Meds: Begin	HCTZ[a] (50 mg 1/day)	Prazosin (2 mg 2/day)	0	0	0	0
End	0	0	0	0	0	0
BP (first 2–7 sess.)	167/101	131/79	151/89	132/92	152/97	143/91
BP (last 2–7 sess.)	147/81	128/77	123/72	121/79	125/76	125/75
% Change in BP	−12/−20	−3/−1	−19/−19	−8/−14	−18/−21	−12/−12
mm Hg Change in BP	−20/−20	−3/−2	−28/−17	−11/−13	−27/−21	−18/−16
No. of Sessions	21	20	11	25	8	11

SUCCESSFUL IN PROGRESS

Patient No.	7	8
Age	65	54
Race/Sex/Mar. Status	W/F/M	W/F/M
Meds: Begin	Chlorthalidone (50 mg 1/day)	0
End	Chlorthalidone (50 mg 1/day)	0

(continued on next page)

Table 4. Blood Pressure Data on the First Eighteen Patients Undergoing Transactional Psychophysiology (TP) Therapy, Cont'd.

BP (first 2–7 sess.)	161/96	164/93
BP (last 2–7 sess.)	136/89	135/77
% Change in BP	−15/−7	−17/−18
mm Hg Change in BP	−25/−7	−29/−16
No. of Sessions	48	40

PARTIALLY SUCCESSFUL IN PROGRESS

Patient No.	9	10	11	12	13	14
Age	39	50	30	43	52	53
Race/Sex/Mar. Status	B/M/S	W/M/M	W/M/M	W/M/M	W/M/M	W/M/D
Meds: Begin	0	Methyldopa (250 mg 3/day) Guanethidine (10 mg 1/day) Clonidine (1 mg 2/day)	Propranolol (40 mg 2/day) HCTZ (50 mg 1/day)	Metoprolol (50 mg 2/day) HCTZ (as needed)	Metoprolol (50 mg 2/day)	HCTZ (50 mg 1/day) Apresoline (80 mg 1/day) Nadolol (40 mg 1/day)
End	0	Methyldopa (500 mg 1/day) Atenolol (10 mg 1/day)	Propranolol (40 mg 1/day)	Metoprolol (50 mg 2/day)	Metoprolol (50 mg 2/day)	Atenolol (25 mg 2/day)
BP (first 2–7 sess.)	136/87	142/90	127/78	149/99	146/91	153/93
BP (last 2–7 sess.)	126/80	134/83	134/89	141/90	133/86	134/85
% Change in BP	−7/−8	−6/−8	+6/+15	−5/−9	−8/−5	−12/−8
mm Hg Change in BP	−10/−7	−8/−7	+7/+11	−8/−9	−13/−5	−19/−8
No. of Sessions	18	10	21	55	51	31

IN PROGRESS REFRACTORY

Patient No.	*15*
Age	60
Race/Sex/Mar. Status	W/M/M
Meds: Begin	Clonidine (.8 mg 1/day)
	HCTZ (50 mg 1/day)
End	Clonidine (.8 mg 1/day)
	HCTZ (50 mg 1/day)
BP (first 2–7 sess.)	148/93
BP (last 2–7 sess.)	151/101
% Change in BP	+2/+8
mm Hg Change in BP	+3/+8
No. of Sessions	58

DROPOUT SUCCESSFUL

Patient No.	*16*
Age	42
Race/Sex/Mar. Status	W/M/M
Meds: Begin	HCTZ (100 mg 1/day)
End	HCTZ (50 mg 1/day)

(continued on next page)

Table 4. Blood Pressure Data on the First Eighteen Patients Undergoing Transactional Psychophysiology (TP) Therapy, Cont'd.

BP (first 2–7 sess.)	148/96
BP (last 2–7 sess.)	140/90
% Change in BP	–5/–6
mm Hg Change in BP	–8/–6
No. of Sessions	11

DROPOUT PARTIALLY SUCCESSFUL

Patient No.	*17*	*18*
Age	59	51
Race/Sex/Mar. Status	W/F/M	W/F/M
Meds: Begin	0	Spironolactone (25 mg 2–3/day)
End	0	Spironolactone (25 mg 2–3/day)
BP (first 2–7 sess.)	162/97	157/100
BP (last 2–7 sess.)	152/90	153/93
% Change in BP	–6/–8	–2/–7
mm Hg Change in BP	–10/–7	–4/–7
No. of Sessions	6	7

[a]Hydrochlorothiazide.

References

Agras, W. S. "Relaxation Therapy in Hypertension." *Hospital Practice,* May 1983, pp. 129-137.

Agras, W. S., Southam, M. A., and Taylor, C. B. "Long-Term Predictors of Relaxation-Induced Blood Pressure Lowering During the Work Day." *Journal of Consulting and Clinical Psychology,* 1983, *51,* 192-194.

Agras, W. S., and others. "Relaxation Training." *Archives of General Psychiatry,* 1980, *37,* 859-863.

Alexander, F. "Psychoanalytic Study of a Case of Essential Hypertension." *Psychosomatic Medicine,* 1939, *1,* 139-156.

Ames, R. P., and Hill, P. "Elevation of Serum Lipid Levels During Diuretic Therapy of Hypertension." *American Journal of Medicine,* 1976, *61,* 748-757.

Bali, L. R. "Long-Term Effect of Relaxation on Blood Pressure and Anxiety Levels of Essential Hypertensive Males: A Controlled Study." *Psychosomatic Medicine,* 1979, *41,* 637-646.

Beiman, I., Graham, L. E., and Ciminero, A. R. "Self-Control Progressive Relaxation Training as an Alternative Nonpharmacological Treatment for Essential Hypertension: Therapeutic Effects in the Natural Environment." *Behaviour Research and Therapy,* 1978, *16,* 371-375.

Benson, H., Marzetta, B. R., and Rosner, B. A. "Decreased Blood Pressure Associated with the Regular Elicitation of the Relaxation Response: A Study of Hypertensive Subjects." In R. S. Eliot (Ed.), *Contemporary Problems in Cardiology.* Vol. 1: *Stress and the Heart.* Mt. Kisco, N.Y.: Futura, 1974.

Benson, H., and Wallace, R. K. "Decreased Blood Pressure in Hypertensive Subjects Who Practice Meditation." *Circulation,* 1972, *46* (supp. II), 130.

Benson, H., and others. "Decreased Systolic Blood Pressure Through Operant Conditioning Techniques in Patients with Essential Hypertension." *Science,* 1971, *173,* 740-742.

Benson, H., and others. "Decreased Blood Pressure in Borderline Hypertensive Patients Who Practice Meditation." *Journal of Chronic Diseases,* 1974a, *27,* 163-169.

Benson, H., and others. "Decreased Blood Pressure in Pharmacologically Treated Hypertensive Patients Who Regularly Elicited the Relaxation Response." *Lancet,* 1974b, *1,* 289-291.

Bertilson, H. S., Bartz, A. E., and Zimmerman, A. D. "Treatment Program for Borderline Hypertension Among College Students: Relaxation, Finger Temperature Biofeedback, and Generalization." *Psychological Reports,* 1979, *44,* 107-114.

Blackwell, B., and others. "Transcendental Meditation in Hypertension." *Lancet,* 1976, *1,* 223-226.

Blanchard, E. B., Young, L. D., and Haynes, M. R. "A Simple Feedback System for the Treatment of Elevated Blood Pressure." *Behavior Therapy,* 1975, *6,* 241-245.

Blanchard, E. B., and others. "Evaluation of Biofeedback in the Treatment of Borderline Essential Hypertension." *Journal of Applied Behavior Analysis,* 1979, *12,* 99-109.

Brady, J. P., Luborsky, L., and Kron, R. E. "Blood Pressure Reduction in Patients with Essential Hypertension Through Metronome-Conditioned Relaxation: A Preliminary Report." *Behavior Therapy,* 1974, *5,* 203-209.

Brandt, E. "Assistant Secretary for Health's Advisory on Treatment of Mild Hypertension." FDA *Drug Bulletin,* 1983, *13,* 24-25.

Cannon, W. B. *Bodily Changes in Pain, Hunger, Fear, and Rage.* New York: Appleton-Century-Croft, 1929.

Christoph, P., and others. "Blood Pressure, Heart Rate, and Respiratory Responses to a Single Session of Relaxation: A Partial Replication." *Journal of Psychosomatic Research,* 1978, *22,* 493-501.

Cohen, P. H. "Analysis of the Final Common Path for Heart Rate Conditioning." In P. A. Obrist and others (Eds.), *Cardiovascular Psychophysiology: Current Issues in Response Mechanisms, Biofeedback, and Methodology.* Hawthorne, N.Y.: Aldine, 1974.

Crowther, J. "Stress Management Training and Relaxation Imagery in the Treatment of Essential Hypertension." *Journal of Behavioral Medicine,* 1983, *6,* 169-187.

Datey, K. K., and others. " 'Shavasan': A Yogic Exercise in the Management of Hypertension." *Angiology,* 1969, *20,* 325-333.

Deabler, H. L., Fidel, E., and Dillenkoffer, R. L. "The Use of Relaxation and Hypnosis in Lowering High Blood Pressure." *American Journal of Clinical Hypnosis,* 1973, *16,* 75-83.

DiCara, L. V., and Miller, N. E. "Instrumental Learning of Systolic Blood Pressure Responses by Curarized Rats: Dissociation of Cardiac and Vascular Changes." *Psychosomatic Medicine,* 1978, *40,* 489-494.

Duke, M. "Thiazide Induced Hypokalemia Association with Acute Myocardial Infarction and Ventricular Fibrillation." *Journal of the American Medical Association,* 1978, *239,* 43-45.

Dykman, R. A., Gantt, W. H., and Whitehorn, J. C. "Conditioning as Emotional Sensitization and Differentiation." *Psychological Monographs,* 1956, *70* (whole No. 15).

Elder, S. T., and Eustis, N. K. "Instrumental Blood Pressure Conditioning in Out-Patient Hypertensives." *Behaviour Research and Therapy,* 1975, *13,* 185-188.

Elder, S. T., and others. "Instrumental Conditioning of Diastolic Blood Pressure in Essential Hypertensive Patients." *Journal of Applied Behavior Analysis,* 1973, *6,* 377-382.

Engel, B. T., Glasglow, M. S., and Gaarder, K. R. "Behavioral Treatment of High Blood Pressure: Follow-Up Results and Treatment Recommendations." *Psychosomatic Medicine,* 1983, *45,* 23-29.

Frankel, B. L., and others. "Treatment of Hypertension with Biofeedback and Relaxation Techniques." *Psychosomatic Medicine,* 1978, *40,* 276-293.

Friedman, H., and Taub, H. A. "The Use of Hypnosis and Biofeedback Procedures for Essential Hypertension." *International Journal of Clinical and Experimental Hypnosis,* 1977, *25,* 335-347.

Friedmann, E., and others. "The Effects of Normal and Rapid Speech on Blood Pressure." *Psychosomatic Medicine,* 1982, *44,* 545-553.

Gantt, W. H. *Experimental Basis for Neurotic Behavior.* New York: Agathon Press, 1944.

Gantt, W. H. "Cardiovascular Components of the Conditional Reflex to Pain, Food, and Other Stimuli." *Physiological Review,* 1960, *40,* 266-291.

Gantt, W. H. "Pavlovian, Classical Conditional Reflex—A Classical Error?" *Conditional Reflex,* 1967a, *2,* 255-257.

Gantt, W. H. "Schizokinesis and Fractional Conditioning." *Conditional Reflex,* 1967b, *2,* 85-87.

Gantt, W. H., and Hoffman, W. C. "Conditioned Cardio-Respiratory Changes Accompanying Conditioned Food Reflexes." *American Journal of Psychology,* 1940, *129,* 360-361.

Goldman, H., and others. "Relationship Between Essential Hypertension and Cognitive Functioning: Effects of Biofeedback." *Psychophysiology,* 1975, *12,* 569-573.

Graham, D. T., Kabler, J. D., and Graham, F. K. "Experimental Production of Predicted Physiological Differences by Suggestion of Attitude." *Psychosomatic Medicine,* 1960, *22,* 321.

Graham, D. T., Kabler, J. D., and Graham, F. K. "Physiological Response to the Suggestion of Attitudes Specific for Hives and Hypertension." *Psychosomatic Medicine,* 1962, *24,* 159-169.

Graham, F. K. "Specific Attitudes in Initial Interviews with Patients Having Different Psychosomatic Diseases." *Psychosomatic Medicine,* 1962, *24,* 257-266.

Green, E. E., Green, A. M., and Norris, P. A. "Preliminary Observations on a New Method for Control of Hypertension." *Journal of the South Carolina Medical Association,* 1979, *75,* 575-582.

Hall, P. S., and others. "Measurement of Neonatal Blood Pressure: A New Method." *Psychophysiology,* 1982, *19,* 231-236.

Harshfield, G. A., and others. "Situational Variations of Blood Pressure in Ambulatory Hypertensive Patients." *Psychosomatic Medicine,* 1982, *44,* 237-245.

Holland, O. B., and others. "Diuretic-Induced Ventricular Ectopic Activity." *American Journal of Medicine,* 1981, *70,* 762-768.

Hollifield, J. W., and Slaton, P. E. "Cardiac Arrhythmias Associated with Diuretic-Induced Hypokalemia and Hypomagnesemia." In C. Wood and W. Somerville (Eds.), *Arrythmia and Myocardial Infarction: The Role of Potassium.* London: Royal Society of Medicine, 1981.

Hypertension Detection and Follow-Up Program Cooperative

Group. "Five Year Findings of the Hypertension Detection and Follow-Up Program. I: Reduction in Mortality of Persons with High Blood Pressure, Including Mild Hypertension." *Journal of the American Medical Association,* 1979, *242,* 2572-2577.

Jacob, R. G., Kraemer, H. C., and Agras, W. S. "Relaxation Therapy in the Treatment of Hypertension: A Review." *Archives of General Psychiatry,* 1977, *34,* 1417-1427.

Jacobson, E. "Use of Relaxation in Hypertensive States." *New York Medical Journal,* 1920, *111,* 419-426.

Jacobson, E. "Variation of Blood Pressure with Skeletal Muscle Tension and Relaxation." *Annals of Internal Medicine,* 1939, *12,* 1194-1212.

Kaplan, N. M. "The Control of Hypertension: A Therapeutic Breakthrough." *American Scientist,* 1980, *68,* 537-545.

Kesteloot, H., and Joossens, J. U. (Eds.). *Epidemiology of Arterial Blood Pressure.* Hingham, Mass.: Kluwer Boston, 1980.

Kleinman, K. M., and others. "Relationship Between Essential Hypertension and Cognitive Functioning. II: Effects of Biofeedback Training Generalize to Non-Laboratory Environment." *Psychophysiology,* 1977, *14,* 192-197.

Klumbies, G., and Eberhardt, G. "Results of Autogenic Training in the Treatment of Hypertension." In J. J. Ibor (Ed.), *IV World Congress of Psychiatry.* International Congress Series, No. 117. Amsterdam: Excerpta Medica Foundation, 1966.

Kristt, D. A., and Engel, B. T. "Learned Control of Blood Pressure in Patients with High Blood Pressure." *Circulation,* 1975, *51,* 370-378.

Long, J. M., and others. "The Effect of Status on Blood Pressure During Verbal Communication." *Journal of Behavioral Medicine,* 1982, *5,* 165-172.

Luborsky, L., and others. "Behavioral Versus Pharmacological Treatments for Essential Hypertension—A Needed Comparison." *Psychosomatic Medicine,* 1982, *44,* 203-213.

Luthe, W. *Autogenic Therapy.* (6 vols.) New York: Grune & Stratton, 1969.

Lynch, J. J. "The Stimulus—The Ghost—The Response: The Carousel of Conditioning." *Conditional Reflex,* 1970, *5,* 133-139.

Lynch, J. J. "Biofeedback: Some Reflections in Modern Behavioral Science." In L. Birk (Ed.), *Biofeedback and Behavioral Medicine*. New York: Grune & Stratton, 1973.

Lynch, J. J. *The Broken Heart: The Medical Consequences of Loneliness*. New York: Harper & Row, 1979.

Lynch, J. J., and others. "Human Speech and Blood Pressure." *Journal of Nervous and Mental Disease*, 1980, *168*, 526-534.

Lynch, J. J., and others. "The Effects of Talking on the Blood Pressure of Hypertensive and Normotensive Individuals." *Psychosomatic Medicine*, 1981, *43*, 25-33.

Lynch, J. J., and others. "Blood Pressure Changes While Talking." *Israeli Journal of Medical Science*, 1982a, *18*, 575-579.

Lynch, J. J., and others. "Interpersonal Aspects of Blood Pressure Control." *Journal of Nervous and Mental Disease*, 1982b, *170*, 143-153.

Malinow, K. L., and others. "Automated Blood Pressure Recording: The Phenomenon of Blood Pressure Elevations During Speech." *Angiology*, 1982, *33*, 474-479.

Miller, N. E. "Learning of Visceral and Glandular Responses." *Science*, 1969, *163*, 434-445.

Miller, N. E., and Dworkin, B. R. "Critical Issues in Therapeutic Applications of Biofeedback." In G. E. Schwartz and J. Beatty (Eds.), *Biofeedback: Theory and Research*. New York: Academic Press, 1977.

Moses, L., Daniels, G. E., and Nickerson, J. L. "Psychogenic Factors in Essential Hypertension." *Psychosmatic Medicine*, 1956, *18* (6), 471-485.

Multiple Risk Factor Intervention Trial Research Group. "Multiple Risk Factor Intervention, Dual Risk Factor Changes, and Mortality Results." *Journal of the American Medical Association*, 1982, *248*, 1465-1477.

Obrist, P. A. "The Cardiovascular-Behavioral Interaction as It Appears Today." *Psychophysiology*, 1976, *13*, 95-107.

Obrist, P. A., and others. "The Cardiac-Somatic Relationship: Some Reformulations." *Psychophysiology*, 1970, *6*, 569-587.

Obrist, P. A., and others. "Alterations in the Cardiac Contractility During Classical Aversive Conditioning in Dogs: Methodological and Theoretical Implications." *Psychophysiology,* 1972, *9,* 246-261.

Obrist, P. A., and others. "The Cardiac-Somatic Interaction." In P. A. Obrist and others (Eds.), *Cardiovascular Psychophysiology: Current Issues in Response Mechanisms, Biofeedback, and Methodology.* Hawthorne, N.Y.: Aldine, 1974.

Obrist, P. A., and others. "The Relationship Among Heart Rate, Carotid dP/dt, and Blood Pressure in Humans as a Function of the Type of Stress." *Psychophysiology,* 1978, *15,* 102-115.

Obrist, P. A., and others. "Blood Pressure Control Mechanisms and Stress: Implications for the Etiology of Hypertension." In G. Onesti and C. R. Klimt (Eds.), *Hypertension: Determinants, Complications, and Interventions.* New York: Grune & Stratton, 1979.

Patel, C. "Yoga and Biofeedback in the Management of Hypertension." *Lancet,* 1973, *2,* 1053-1055.

Patel, C. "12 Month Follow-Up of Yoga and Biofeedback in the Management of Hypertension." *Lancet,* 1975a, *1,* 62-64.

Patel, C. "Yoga and Biofeedback in the Management of Hypertension." *Journal of Psychosomatic Research,* 1975b, *19,* 355-360.

Patel, C., and Datey, K. K. "Relaxation and Biofeedback Techniques in the Management of Hypertension." *Angiology,* 1976, *27,* 106-113.

Patel, C., Marmot, M. G., and Terry, D. J. "Controlled Trial of Biofeedback-Aided Behavioral Methods in Reducing Mild Hypertension." *British Medical Journal,* 1981, *282,* 2005-2008.

Patel, C., and North, W. R. S. "Randomised Controlled Trial of Yoga and Biofeedback in Management of Hypertension." *Lancet,* 1975, *2,* 93-95.

Patel, D. J., and others. "A Control Procedure for Studies of Blood Pressure Feedback in Hypertension." *Cardiovascular Medicine,* 1978, *3,* 627-630.

Pavlov, I. *Conditioned Reflexes: An Investigation of the Physiological Activity of the Cerebral Cortex.* (G. V. Anrep, Trans.) New York: Dover, 1960. (Originally published 1927.)

Pavlov, I. P. "Reply of a Physiologist to Psychologists." *Psychological Review,* 1932, *39,* 91-129.

Pickering, T. G., and others. "Ambulatory Monitoring in the Evaluation of Blood Pressure in Patients with Borderline Hypertension and the Role of the Defense Reflex." *Clinical and Experimental Hypertension,* 1982a, *A4,* 675-693.

Pickering, T. G., and others. "Blood Pressure During Normal Daily Activities, Sleep, and Exercise: Comparison of Values in Normal and Hypertensive Subjects." *Journal of the American Medical Association,* 1982b, *247,* 992-996.

Pollack, A. A., and others. "Limitations of Transcendental Meditation in the Treatment of Essential Hypertension." *Lancet,* 1977, *1,* 71-73.

"Race, Education, and Prevalence of Hypertension: Hypertension Detection and Follow-Up Group in America." *Journal of Epidemiology,* 1977, *106,* 351-359.

Redmond, D. P., and others. "Blood Pressure and Heart Rate Response to Verbal Instructions and Relaxation in Hypertension." *Psychosomatic Medicine,* 1974, *36,* 285-297.

Reichgott, M. J., and Simons-Morton, B. G. "Strategies to Improve Patient Compliance with Antihypertensive Therapy." *Primary Care,* 1983, *10,* 21-27.

Reiser, M. F., and others. "Life Situations, Emotions, and the Course of Patients with Arterial Hypertension." *Psychosomatic Medicine,* 1951, *13* (3), 133-139.

Rescorla, R. A., and Solomon, R. L. "Two Process Learning Theory: Relationships Between Pavlovian Conditioning and Instrumental Learning." *Psychological Review,* 1967, *74,* 151-182.

Rosenman, R. H., and others. "A Predictive Study of Coronary Heart Disease." *Journal of the American Medical Association,* 1964, *189,* 103-110.

Seer, P. "Psychological Control of Essential Hypertension: Review of the Literature and Methodological Critique." *Psychological Bulletin,* 1979, *86* (5), 1015-1043.

Shapiro, A. P., and others. "Relationships of Perception, Cognition, Suggestion, and Operant Conditioning in Essential Hypertension." *Brain Research,* 1975, *312,* 299-312.

Shapiro, A. P., and others. "Behavioral Methods in the Treatment of Hypertension: A Review of Their Clinical Status." *Annals of Internal Medicine,* 1977, *85,* 626-635.

Shapiro, D., and Goldstein, I. B. "Biobehavioral Perspectives on Hypertension." *Journal of Consulting and Clinical Psychology,* 1982, *50* (6), 841-848.

Shoemaker, J. E., and Tasto, D. L. "The Effects of Muscle Relaxation on Blood Pressure of Essential Hypertensives." *Behaviour Research and Therapy,* 1975, *13,* 29-43.

Smith, O. A., and Stebbins, W. C. "Conditioned Blood Flow and Heart Rate in Monkeys." *Journal of Comparative and Physiological Psychology,* 1965, *59,* 432-436.

Smith, W. M., Johnson, W., and Bromer, L. "Intervention Trial in Mild Hypertension." In O. Paul (Ed.), *Epidemiology and Control of Hypertension.* Miami: Symposia Specialists, 1975.

Southam, M. A., and others. "Relaxation Training." *Archives of General Psychiatry,* 1982, *39,* 715-717.

Sterling, P., and Eyer, J. "Biological Basis for Stress Related Mortality." *Social Science and Medicine,* 1981, *15E,* 3-42.

Stone, R. A., and DeLeo, J. "Psychotherapeutic Control of Hypertension." *New England Journal of Medicine,* 1976, *294,* 80-84.

Surwit, R. S., Shapiro, D., and Good, M. I. "Comparison of Cardiovascular Biofeedback, Neuromuscular Biofeedback, and Meditation in the Treatment of Borderline Essential Hypertension." *Journal of Consulting and Clinical Psychology,* 1978, *46,* 252-263.

Taylor, C. B., and others. "Relaxation Therapy and High Blood Pressure." *Archives of General Psychiatry,* 1977, *34,* 339-342.

Thaler, M., Weiner, H., and Reiser, M. F. "Exploration of the Doctor-Patient Relationship Through Projective Techniques." *Psychosomatic Medicine,* 1957, *19,* 228-239.

Thomas, S., and others. "Blood Pressure and Heart Rate Changes in Children While Reading Out Loud in School." *Journal of Public Health Reports,* 1984a, *99,* 77-84.

Thomas, S., and others. "Changes in Nurses' Blood Pressure and Heart Rate While Communicating." *Journal of Research in Nursing and Health,* 1984b, *7,* 119-126.

United States Public Health Service Hospitals Cooperative

Study Group. "Morbidity and Mortality in Mild Essential Hypertension." *Circulation Research* (supp. II), 1972, *30* and *31*, 11-110 and 11-124.

Veterans Administration Cooperative Study Group on Antihypertensive Agents. "Effects of Treatment on Morbidity in Hypertension: Results in Patients with Diastolic Pressure Averaging 115 Through 129 mm Hg." *Journal of the American Medical Association,* 1967, *202,* 1028-1034.

Veterans Administration Cooperative Study Group on Antihypertensive Agents. "Effects of Treatment on Morbidity in Hypertension: Results in Patients with Diastolic Pressure Averaging 90 Through 114 mm Hg." *Journal of the American Medical Association,* 1970, *213,* 1143-1152.

Veterans Administration Cooperative Study Group on Antihypertensive Agents. "Effects of Treatment on Morbidity in Hypertension: Influence of Age, Diastolic Pressure, and Prior Cardiovascular Disease: Further Analysis of Side Effects." *Circulation,* 1972, *45,* 173-186.

Walsh, P., Dale, A., and Anderson, D. E. "Comparison of Biofeedback Pulse Wave Velocity and Progressive Relaxation in Essential Hypertensives." *Perceptual and Motor Skills,* 1977, *44,* 839-843.

Weiner, H. *Psychobiology of Essential Hypertension.* New York: Elsevier, 1979.

Wolf, S., and Wolff, H. G. "A Summary of Experimental Evidence Relating Life Stress to the Pathogenesis of Essential Hypertension in Man." In E. T. Bell (Ed.), *Essential Hypertension.* Minneapolis: University of Minnesota Press, 1951.

Wolf, S., and others. *Life Stress and Essential Hypertension.* Baltimore: Williams & Wilkens, 1955.

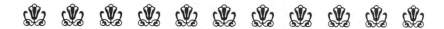

2

Arrhythmias: Evaluating and Managing Problems of Heart Rate and Rhythm

Michael Feuerstein, *Ph.D.*
Ronald Cohen, *Ph.D.*

Biobehavioral factors have long been thought to play a role in the etiology, exacerbation, and/or maintenance of certain types of cardiac arrhythmias. Consequently, techniques such as biofeedback, relaxation training, meditation, hypnosis, and psychotherapy have been used in the management of certain patients with cardiac arrhythmias. The aim of this chapter is to review (1) the pathophysiology and etiology of cardiac arrhythmias, integrating biobehavioral factors; (2) the biobehavioral evaluation

Portions of the "Review of Treatment Literature" section were adapted from Feuerstein and Ward (1980). We express our gratitude to Gary Gefken for his assistance with the case material presented.

of the patient with arrhythmias; and (3) biobehavioral approaches to the management of cardiac arrhythmias.

Therapists without medical training who use biobehavioral approaches tend to consider arrhythmias as a single undifferentiated phenomenon or as an entity independent of any underlying disease process. Both of these notions are largely inaccurate. Cardiac arrhythmias, in fact, represent a broad heterogeneous class of syndromes characterized by electrical disturbances of the heart and are usually manifested as abnormalities of rate, rhythm, or conductive pattern. Furthermore, although certain types of arrhythmias are common in normal individuals or individuals without obvious organic pathology, many arrhythmias result from a variety of disease processes that produce either a structural or a biochemical abnormality of conduction in cardiac tissue (Bellet, 1971). It is therefore important to review briefly the various types of arrhythmias, along with their different etiologies and mechanisms.

Consideration of the classification of arrhythmias reveals a complex picture. While it is beyond the scope of this chapter to discuss each of the variants of arrhythmias, a discussion of certain taxonomies will be presented. Arrhythmias have been traditionally classified according to anatomical location in the heart, type of disturbance in rhythm (for example, tachycardia), and/or underlying mechanisms. Classification of underlying mechanisms includes disorders due to impulse formation, impulse conduction, or both impulse formation and conduction (Bigger, 1980). Impulse formation disorders generally disrupt the mechanisms of automaticity, while impulse conduction disorders usually involve the reentry of impulses. Reentry is defined as a process by which a cardiac impulse is forced to take an alternative and usually longer pathway because of a block in a normal pathway.

Cardiac arrhythmias are classified and defined by both the nature of the disturbance in beat and the anatomical location of the disorder. Table 1 contains a classification scheme of various arrhythmias occurring at different anatomical sites. As can be seen from this classification, arrhythmias involve various

Table 1. Classification of Arrhythmias.

Disturbances of Rhythm Involving the Sinoatrial Node
Sinus arrhythmia
Sinus bradycardia
Sinoatrial block
Prolonged sinus pauses
Wandering pacemaker
Sinus tachycardia

Disturbances Involving the Atria
Atrial premature beats
Atrial paroxysmal tachycardia
Atrial flutter
Atrial fibrillation
Intra-atrial block: Intra-atrial dissociation
Atrial standstill
Sinoventricular conduction

Disturbances Involving the Atrioventricular (A-V) Junction
A-V heart block
A-V junctional rhythm
A-V junctional escape, including coronary sinus rhythm
A-V junctional premature beats
Paroxysmal junctional tachycardia
Atrioventricular dissociation
Reciprocal rhythm

Disturbances Involving the Ventricles
Ventricular escape
Idioventricular rhythm
Ventricular premature beats
Ventricular paroxysmal tachycardia
Ventricular flutter and ventricular fibrillation
Cardiac (ventricular) arrest
Heart alternation

From Samuel Bellet, *Clinical Disorders of the Heart Beat* (3rd ed.), (Philadelphia: Lea & Febiger, 1971). Reprinted with permission.

disturbances in rhythm, including tachycardia (rapid heart beat), bradycardia (slow heart beat), and disturbances involving unique beat productions. Disorders of beat production include fibrillation, flutter, and premature beats. The locations of arrhythmias include the sinoatrial node, the atria, the atrioventricular (A-V) junction, and the ventricles.

Underlying Mechanisms and Pathophysiology

The fundamental mechanism underlying normal cardiac activity and impulse conduction is the action potential (Bellet, 1971). When cardiac cells are stimulated, an action potential results. This action potential represents the spreading of electrical current to adjacent cell areas. The electrical current occurs as a result of the cell membrane characteristics of the cardiac muscle. An electrical potential is generated as a result of the relationship between potassium on the inside of the cell membrane and sodium on the outside of the membrane. With the onset of an electrical impulse, a flux occurs as sodium rushes into and across the cell membrane. This results in a depolarization and a rapid spike. Following the depolarization, there is a gradual and then a more rapid repolarization as potassium moves outside of the cell membrane in order to reestablish electrical equilibrium. There are five phases of the cardiac action potential: rapid depolarization, early repolarization, a plateau, rapid repolarization, and a diastolic period. The exact nature of the action potential varies across cell types. For instance, sinoatrial and atrioventricular cells are much slower than Purkinje fibers or atrial and ventricular muscle. The action potential of heart muscle is similar to that occurring in skeletal muscle and nerve cells, though the conduction speed is significantly slower (several hundred msec) compared to the more rapid conduction of nerves. The sequence of the action potential is critical to the maintenance of cardiac rhythm (Trautwein, 1973). Through the action potential, an electrical impulse can be propagated across the heart, producing a set sequence of contractions which ultimately influence the pumping of blood. This sequence of events and associated ECG pattern is illustrated in Figure 1. Interference with this process will result in a disturbance by which impulses are improperly spread across different sites of the heart. Such disturbances are referred to as arrhythmias.

Consideration of the propagation or spreading of the cardiac impulse may facilitate an understanding of how cardiac rhythm may become dysfunctional. The normal cardiac impulse is initiated in specialized T cells of the sinoatrial node. The sino-

Figure 1. Cardiac Conduction Sequence as Reflected on
the ECG. Note That the Impulse Travels from the
Sinoatrial Node to the Atrioventricular Node Down into
the His-Purkinje System and Ventricular Myocardium.

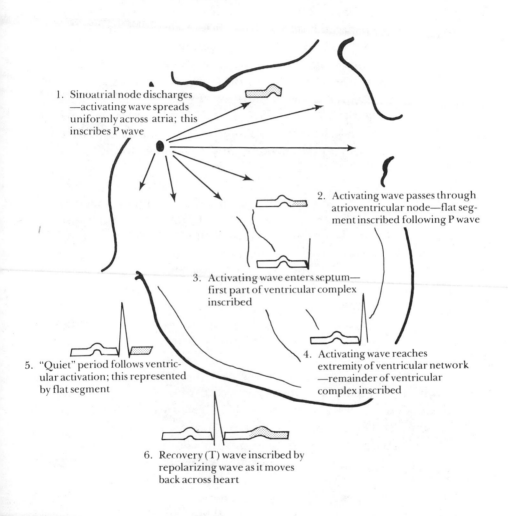

1. Sinoatrial node discharges
   —activating wave spreads
   uniformly across atria; this
   inscribes P wave

2. Activating wave passes through
   atrioventricular node—flat segment inscribed following P wave

3. Activating wave enters septum—
   first part of ventricular complex
   inscribed

4. Activating wave reaches
   extremity of ventricular network
   —remainder of ventricular
   complex inscribed

5. "Quiet" period follows ventricular activation; this represented
   by flat segment

6. Recovery (T) wave inscribed by
   repolarizing wave as it moves
   back across heart

From B. Phibbs, *The Cardiac Arrhythmias* (3rd ed.) (Saint Louis:
Mosby, 1978). Reprinted with permission of the author.

atrial node, located superior to the right atrial wall, contains cells that are capable of automaticity and therefore have a pace-maker function for the heart. Automaticity seems to be medi-ated by catecholamines such that acetylcholine suppresses and norepinephrine increases automatic cardiac activity. Cells of the sinoatrial node appear to have automaticity in part because they undergo depolarization during certain stages of the action potential. Under normal conditions heart rate depends on the degree of automaticity of the sinoatrial cells. Impulses arise from this node at a rate between 60 and 140 beats per minute. Besides the sinoatrial node, cells of the His bundle, the terminal of the Purkinje fibers, the atrioventricular node, and some spe-cialized atrial areas also have capability for automaticity. These areas normally act as pacemakers only as long as normal sinus rhythm prevails.

Following the generation of an impulse from the sino-atrial node, there is a spreading of electrical excitability across transitional cells in the atrium. From the atrium the impulse moves to the atrioventricular junction, the His-Purkinje system, and finally to the ventricular myocardium. The impulse moves at a relatively rapid rate (100 mm/sec) across the atria, then slows to 20 mm/sec in the atrioventricular junction, and finally acceler-ates to its greatest velocity (4,000 mm/sec) in the ventricular Purkinje fibers. These fluctuations in the conduction of the im-pulse through the Purkinje fibers create the conditions for con-traction of the ventricular muscle.

Subcortical brain structures and the autonomic nervous system have important roles in normal cardiovascular function. Lown, Verrier, and Rabinowitz (1977) have specified the hypo-thalamus and quadrigeminal bodies as areas affecting cardiac rhythm. Hypothalamic stimulation can produce arrhythmias and lower the threshold of ventricular vulnerability, making the occurrence of a ventricular contraction more probable. The heart is innervated by both sympathetic and parasympathetic nerves. Cortical arousal may affect these autonomic systems, causing changes in heart rhythm. Therefore, while normal car-diac rhythm is dependent on the action potential and the capac-ity of the various components of the heart to propagate the impulse, factors outside of the cardiovascular system (for example, the central nervous system) may also affect rhythm.

Normal heart rhythm depends on the ability of the various components of the heart to function within an acceptable *sequence,* and on homeostatic mechanisms that maintain this sequence of activation. Various factors, such as genetically determined metabolic needs, may affect the functioning of individual cardiac muscle fibers. Also, such factors as electrolyte imbalances, inflammation, and degenerative processes may inhibit the normal functioning and conduction of the heart. The normal heart serves the body's demand for oxygen and other nutrients via the autonomic nervous system signals that serve to adjust cardiac output. Sympathetic stimulation enhances the contractibility of the heart and the automaticity of the sinoatrial node. Parasympathetic activity exerts the opposite affect. Normal functioning of the myocardium depends on four inherent properties: automaticity, excitability, conductivity, and contractility.

Automaticity, as mentioned earlier, is normally maintained through the sinoatrial node. If the function of this pacemaker is depressed, other automatic tissue of the heart will take over this function at a less efficient rate. In abnormal states groups of cells override the pacemaker function of the sinus node. When this phenomenon occurs, an *ectopic beat or rhythm* is produced. By definition, ectopic refers to the generation of a rhythm from an area outside the sinoatrial node. Increased automaticity in all pacemaker cells may be produced through increased sympathetic activity, decreased parasympathetic activity, decreased potassium, increased calcium, hypercapnia, acidosis, hypoxia, hyperthermia, mechanical effects such as stressing of the muscle, and certain drugs (Bellet, 1971). Decreased automaticity is produced by the reverse set of conditions. In addition, decreased carbon dioxide or increased oxygen in the partial pressure of the blood may reduce automaticity.

Excitability refers to the condition that allows cardiovascular tissue to respond when stimulated. Both increased and decreased excitability are influenced by the relationship of sympathetic to parasympathetic tone. In addition, the absence of

potassium may increase excitability, while its excess may decrease excitability. The depression of automaticity also serves
to increase excitability of the heart. A variety of drugs have the
effect of either increasing or inhibiting the excitability of heart
muscle. When the heart is more excitable, it is likely to show
greater responses of beat production relative to nervous stimulation. In cases of low excitability, stimulation fails to elicit a
response. The role of autonomic and central nervous system factors is evident here. Excitable heart muscle is likely to respond
with *extra beats* or a *faster rate of beat* to ongoing stimulation.

The ability of the tissue of the heart to propagate an impulse from cell to cell is referred to as *conductivity*. Conductivity is related to the excitability of the tissue in question. As
mentioned earlier, different areas of the heart have different ef-
ficiencies for conduction, which result in varying conduction
speeds. In normal heart action, these different speeds of conduction contribute to the normal rhythm. Besides autonomic
nervous system factors and the effects of potassium and calcium, conductivity is influenced by the morphology and health
of the myocardium. Diseases affecting the heart muscle may result in a failure to conduct impulses properly. In the case of
heart block, a structural lesion results in a failure of conduction along normal pathways.

Contractility refers to the ability of heart muscle to contract and ultimately to pump blood in response to impulses generated throughout the heart. The metabolic requirements of the
myocardium, particularly with respect to adenosine triphos-
phate (ATP) and calcium in the sarcoplasmic reticulum of the
cell, seem to affect the ability of the heart muscle to contract.
Abnormalities in this metabolism—as a result of anemia, hypothermia, hyperthyroidism, or hypercalcemia—may increase the
heart's contraction. Emotions and exercise also seem to increase
contractility. Contractility is decreased as a function of long
periods of rest, myocardial disease, hypothyroidism, hypocal-
cemia, and certain shock-like states. Again, various drugs may
also affect contractility.

Disturbances of either impulse formation or conduction
result from abnormalities in the four properties mentioned

above. Disturbances of impulse formation that affect automaticity usually occur when sinoatrial node efficiency is depressed. At these times other potential pacemakers in the transitional atrial tracts and His-Purkinje systems assume primary function, resulting in the ectopic beats.

Disturbances of conduction occur in response to various abnormalities in the atria, the atrioventricular junction, or throughout the ventricles. Normal conduction time is increased when, because of a block, the impulse has to travel over abnormal pathways. When conduction is delayed, impulses may arrive during periods of the action potential that are not suitable for excitation. As a result, a subsequent action potential may occur with abnormal characteristics. The reentry of cardiac impulses occurs when alternate pathways of conduction are followed because of blocks in normal pathways. Such blocks may occur at either the atrioventricular node or locally at various sites in the myocardium. Different arrhythmias result according to the anatomical site of the block. Often it is difficult to distinguish between disorders of reentry and disorders of automaticity. Heart blocks at the A-V junction affect the rate of depolarization, and automaticity therefore becomes enhanced in the Purkinje fibers. The automaticity of the Purkinje fibers ultimately affects conduction through them. Certain arrhythmias are characterized by close interaction between disorders of impulse formation and conduction. In a common type of combined arrhythmia (the parasystole), one or more ectopic areas begin to fire and act as pacemakers in addition to the sinoatrial node. In the parasystole reentry occurs because normal impulse from the sinoatrial node does not pass through this new ectopic area. A disorder of automaticity also occurs, since the parasystole also acts as pacemaker.

Several regulatory mechanisms are often subject to dysfunction in arrhythmias. These include physical regulation of blood flow, autonomic nervous system regulation, regulation of metabolism, and endocrine regulation. The physical regulation of blood flow is important, since the heart functions in a pressure-volume relationship. As blood pressure changes, cardiac metabolism and electrolyte balances also change. Changes in pressure also result in possible stretching of myocardial fibers, and an arrhythmia may result.

As mentioned earlier, the nervous system has very direct regulatory control over the heart. At a central level, besides the hypothalamus, the cerebral cortex, the vasomotor center of the fourth ventricle, the basal ganglia, and the medullary vagal nuclei also exhibit cardiovascular control functions. A variety of internal and external stimuli may influence the excitability of these areas. The limbic system contains pathways into the midbrain, which ultimately influences the medulla. Therefore, emotional factors seem to impinge ultimately on cardiovascular regulation. The sympathetic and parasympathetic effects on automaticity, excitability, and conductivity of impulses have already been discussed.

Metabolic products, such as hydrogen, lactate, carbon dioxide, ATP, and histamine, control regional blood flow and also influence the neural and reflex control mechanisms of the heart. Endocrine substances, such as aldosterone, exert influence on the kidney, which ultimately affects cardiovascular activity. The adrenocorticotropic hormone influences cortisol, which affects the reactivity of smooth muscle in response to neurotransmitters. Diseases of the thyroid also affect endocrine function and may result in cardiovascular arrhythmias.

Finally, pathological factors may produce arrhythmias. These factors include ischemic changes (due to infarction and a loss of blood flow to a particular region for a period of time) and inflammatory diseases affecting the heart. Both factors may result in lesions affecting various anatomic locations in the heart, and may ultimately result in a blocked conduction pathway, which will lead to an arrhythmia.

Etiology and Prevalence

The incidence of cardiac arrhythmias is dependent on numerous factors relative to the population studied. Specifically, the age and medical status of the patient group being observed will influence the types of arrhythmias observed. Also, the method of assessment influences incidence, since certain arrhythmias may be more prevalent when observed under special conditions (such as ambulatory recording). Nonetheless, a few studies have documented relative incidences of the various arrhythmias in rather large patient groups over extended time periods.

Katz and Pick (1956) studied 50,000 patients over a twenty-five-year period. The most frequently observed arrhythmias were those of premature beats (14.5 percent). Atrial fibrillation occurred in 11.7 percent of patients; A-V heart block in 4.2 percent; A-V dissociation in 1.4 percent; and atrial flutter in .5 percent. Only 35 percent of the cases showed normal sinus rhythm, while 20 percent had sinus tachycardia, bradycardia, or other such irregularities. In another study Ostrander and associates (1965) studied the electrocardiograms of 5,129 general, nonhospitalized adults in a single town and found first-degree A-V block in 1.4 percent, frequent premature contractions in 1.9 percent, incomplete left bundle branch block in 1.4 percent, A-V junctional rhythm in .6 percent, atrial fibrillations in .4 percent, and complete bundle branch blocks in .4 percent of the sample. While most arrhythmias are associated with particular disease processes, many arrhythmias occur in a percentage of normal patients. For instance, 5-10 percent of individuals with paroxysmal ventricular tachycardia show no evidence of organic heart disease (Fowler, 1980).

A common site of arrhythmias is the sinoatrial node. Disorders of the sinus include tachycardia, bradycardia, wandering atrial pacemaker, and sinoatrial block. Sick sinus syndrome—a sinus arrhythmia of the sinus node activation and impulse conduction—results in sinus bradycardia, which in turn often results in intermittent atrial tachycardia. Sinus node arrest or sinoatrial block (Ferrer, 1973), another type of sinoatrial arrhythmia, is found with a variety of conditions, including vagal stimulation, catecholamine depletion, metabolic disorders such as hypothyroidism, drug toxicity, and specific diseases of the atria and sinoatrial node. It can also occur in normal, healthy adults, especially athletes. Syncope is a common symptom with this type of arrhythmia.

Sinus bradycardia is thought to occur in 20 percent of patients with acute myocardial infarction and 61 percent of indi-

viduals with inferior wall infarction. Sinus tachycardia may occur in the presence of any sympathetic stimulation—in particular, anxiety, fever, exercise, hyperthyroidism, shock, and congestive heart failure. Most instances of sinus tachycardia are not
related to a disease process.

Premature cardiac contractions, the most common arrhythmia, occur with a wide variety of conditions, including
acute infarction, coronary insufficiency, mitral valve syndrome,
and cardiomyopathies. In this disorder premature "ectopic"
beats arise from any automatic heart tissue. A large number of
patients without heart disease experience this arrhythmia. In
fact, Hinkle, Carver, and Stevens (1969) found that such beats
are very common in patients between fifty and seventy years of
age. Premature ventricular contractions, which commonly precede ventricular fibrillation in acute myocardial infarction,
however, have been considered a serious risk factor for death.

Premature atrial contractions are also frequent, yet rarely
associated with increased mortality. This condition is often
associated with fatigue, anxiety, or intake of substances such as
caffeine or tobacco. Occasionally, when symptoms are bother-
some, treatment is required.

Atrial and atrioventricular tachycardias arise from ectopic
atrial foci and are characterized by regular onset and offset.
These tachycardias are often found in patients with rheumatic,
arteriosclerotic, and hypertensive diseases, as well as in a large
group of normal individuals. The paroxyms are often related to
emotional stress, fatigue, substance intake, and particular syndromes (such as Wolff-Parkinson-White). Nonparoxysmal A-V
tachycardia results from abnormal enhancement of impulse
formation and is associated with severe heart disease (myocar-
ditis and acute myocardial infarction).

Atrial fibrillation is one of the most common arrhythmias
of the heart and is usually associated with diseases that enlarge
the left atrium. Fowler (1980) observed that one third of his
patients with tight mitral stenosis and nonobstructive cardiomyopathies experienced atrial fibrillations. Atrial fibrillation is
found in 10 percent of patients with acute infections, 25 percent with pericarditis, and 10 percent with hyperthyroidism.

Atrial flutter is a rapid, regular, continuous wave movement in the atria and is rarer than atrial fibrillation. Atrial flutter is usually associated with an underlying disease. This arrhythmia is characterized by very high rate (300/min) and a saw-tooth pattern on ECG. The onset of atrial flutter is rapid and is often associated with "heart pounding" or "palpitation."

Ventricular tachycardia is found in 72 percent of patients with coronary artery disease and in 10 percent of patients with infarcts (Bellet, 1971). Digitalis toxicity and rheumatic disease are also common causes. This type of arrhythmia is particularly serious because it results in ineffective cardiac pumping, which may cause shock and pulmonary edema.

Factors Associated with Exacerbation

While cardiac arrhythmias are often associated with specific disease processes, a number of factors seem to trigger or exacerbate their occurrence. For years there have been clinical reports that anxiety, stress, fatigue, coffee, cigarettes, exercise, and food intake can influence the occurrence of arrhythmias. A physiological relationship between these factors and arrhythmias has been assumed (Katz, Winton, and Megibow, 1947), though until recently there was little empirical evidence for such an association. Particular controversy surrounded the question of whether emotional state specifically influences cardiac rhythm (Regestein, 1975).

There now is considerable evidence that psychological stress and anxiety can contribute to arrhythmias (Lown and DeSilva, 1978; Lynch and others, 1977b). Reports from cardiological practices estimate that 10–14 percent of patients experience anxiety-derived cardiac complaints (Fowler, 1980). Anxiety influences cardiovascular control. Sympathetic activity increases the automaticity of the heart through mediation of phase four of the intracellular potential of the sinoatrial node. Cholinergic vagal innervation has been shown to modify the thresholds for ventricular excitability, thereby interacting with sympathetic arousal in influencing arrhythmias (Lown, Verrier, and Corbalan, 1973).

Several studies have demonstrated a relationship between psychological stress, sympathetic activation, and the occurrence of arrhythmias. Lown, Verrier, and Corbalan produced
extrasystoles through the presentation of electric shock to restrained (stress) and unrestrained (no stress) dogs. Extrasystoles
were produced at a lower amperage in the restrained dogs, indicating that the psychological stress associated with restraint had
lowered the threshold for cardiac fibrillation at higher rates in
animals with coronary artery occlusions. These findings suggest
that stress may exacerbate the arrhythmic effects resulting from
structural abnormalities.

Evidence from clinical studies in humans also suggests
that emotional stress affects cardiac rhythm (Hackett and
Rosenbaum, 1980; Lynch and others, 1977b). Automobile driving, public speaking, spectator sports, and other common activities have been shown to alter serum catecholamine levels, resulting in an increased number of ectopic beats. An increased
prevalence of arrhythmias also has been noted during bereave-
ment, suggesting that depressed states may affect cardiac rhythm.
Major life change is often considered a significant stressor, and
evidence suggests that arrhythmias occur more frequently during such periods (Rahe and Romo, 1974). Human contact in the
handling of patients in coronary care units has also been shown
to affect arrhythmias (Lynch and others, 1977a).

In studies of lactate metabolism, exercise tolerance, and
anxiety (Ackerman and Sacher, 1974; Pitts and McClure, 1967),
patients with chronic anxiety were shown to have increased
levels of serum lactate, which was associated with the complex-
ing of calcium ions. A decrease in the binding of calcium to cardiac nerve membranes may lead to symptoms such as palpitations. However, it is unlikely that lactate is the sole basis for
anxiety symptoms, as patients' response to the substance habit-
uates, despite continuance of subjective distress. Hyperactivity
of beta-adrenergic receptors has also been postulated as contributing to these symptoms (Bove, 1977). Behavioral styles and
coping strategies also influence these symptoms, as will be discussed.

There now appears to be considerable evidence that a

Arrhythmias
69

variety of substances produce changes in cardiac rhythm. In particular, cigarettes, coffee, alcohol, and certain medications have been documented to increase arrhythmic activity.

Cigarette smoking has been shown to cause an immediate heart rate acceleration. While the heart rate may diminish following completion of smoking, a temporary sympathetic arousal is often observed (Gilbert and Haggen, 1980). Such an elevation could lower the threshold for arrhythmia in patients with cardiac disturbances. The long-term effects of tobacco intake have been associated with an increased prevalence of cardiac myopathies and coronary artery disease (Jarvik, 1979). Heart blocks produced by these disorders may result in a variety of arrhythmias. Therefore, tobacco intake appears to have both short- and long-term effects on arrhythmias.

Acute coffee ingestion has been associated with the presence of arrhythmias. Dobmeyer and associates (1983) reported sustained atrial flutter-fibrillation, atrioventricular nodal-reentry tachycardia, and ventricular tachycardia (response to ventricular stimulation) following oral caffeine ingestion (200 mg $\simeq$ 2.5 cups) in patients with clinical and echocardiographic evidence of mitral valve prolapse syndrome, cardiomyopathy with cardiomegaly, and symptoms of syncope, near-syncope, and palpitations. Acute administration of caffeine results in a number of physiological changes that can affect cardiac rhythm, including increases in levels of plasma catecholamines, cyclic adinosine-monophosphate (AMP), antidiuretic hormone, and cortical activation. Heavy coffee consumption (nine or more cups a day) in males aged thirty-seven to fifty-seven has been associated with increased risk of ventricular premature beats, in contrast to light consumption (one or two cups a day) or abstinence (Prineas and others, 1980). Coffee consumption therefore should be considered as a potential influence on cardiac arrhythmias.

A variety of psychopharmacological agents also affect cardiac rhythm (Barchas and others, 1977). Specifically, thioridazine is commonly associated with prolonged ventricular repolarization. Other antipsychotics also result in such changes, although less frequently. The tricyclics can result in tachycardia and changes in conduction (prolonged QT intervals, depressed

ST segments, flattened T waves), which may precede onset of ventricular tachyarrhythmias. A number of cardiac medications, in addition to having antiarrhythmic properties, can produce cardiological side effects that may induce arrhythmias. Digitalis is thought to produce toxic side effects in approximately 37 percent of cases. Disruption of cardiac rhythm often accompanies toxicity. A detailed discussion of drug-induced arrhythmias can be found in Braunwald (1980). It should be evident that consideration of the effects of these substances is vital to adequate management of arrhythmias.

Cardiac function is controlled by a complex network of interacting physiological systems (Bellett, 1971). Control of cardiac function is determined by both central and peripheral nervous system components, hormonal influences, mechanical and electrical properties of the heart and circulatory system, and environmental factors. These control systems interact, maintaining a regulated state through an elaborate feedback network.

Disregulation of the cardiovascular system may result from an underlying structural impairment, changes in environmental demands, or changes in the way that environmental demands are internally mediated (for example, changes in hormonal or neurotransmitter levels). In the case of arrhythmias, there may be changes that affect all three factors, and a change in one may ultimately lead to disruption of the other. For instance, an individual experiencing excessive environmental demands may suffer from a myocardial infarction as a result of excessive hypertension. The infarction may result in a heart block, which then causes an arrhythmia. This arrhythmia may be exacerbated by the anxiety or fear of a subsequent myocardial infarction. In other cases there may be a problem in control function; for instance, sinus tachycardia may result from social anxiety without evidence of structural cardiac changes or chronically altered catecholamine levels. Therefore, the clinician working with the arrhythmia patient should determine whether any or all of the control functions are disrupted. The clinician also should determine whether structural abnormality, excessive environmental demands, or exogenous or endogenous biochemical alteration is contributing to the arrhythmia. Such information can be obtained through a comprehensive medical and biobehavioral evaluation. For an overview of issues in this area, the reader is referred to Braunwald (1980).

Evaluation of the Patient with Arrhythmia

As indicated in Table 2, evaluation of the patient with arrhythmia should consist of medical record review; a standard

Table 2. Biobehavioral Assessment of the Patient with Arrhythmia.

Medical Record Review
     History
     Pathophysiological indices
Psychological Interview (Behavior-Analytic)
     Patient's perception of disorder/symptoms
     Coping style
     Levels of anxiety/depression
     Role of stress in exacerbation/maintenance
     Spouse's perception of and response to disorder/symptoms
Psychometric Evaluation
     Psychological characteristics (MMPI: somatization, depression,
       hysterical features, anxiety, activity level)
     Environmental factors of strain (Work Environment Scale, Family
       Environment Scale)
     Illness Behavior (Illness Behavior Questionnaire)
     Potential prognostic indicators of response to biobehavioral
       techniques (Self-Control Schedule, Alexithymia scales)
Ambulatory ECG Monitoring
Health Risk/Lifestyle Appraisal
Biological "Markers" of Melancholia/Depression
     Dexamethasone Suppression Test

---

psychological interview of patient and spouse, if present; psychometric evaluation of psychological characteristics and of environmental (job, family) sources of stress/strain; and other psychological testing as appropriate for a given patient. In select cases a comprehensive evaluation of the roles that various environmental factors may play in exacerbating the arrhythmia(s) should also be undertaken, incorporating ambulatory ECG monitoring. Assessment of health risk/lifestyle factors contributory to cardiovascular disease also proves useful in obtaining a complete picture of the biobehavioral factors associated with the disorder. The clinician should attempt to identify psychological, psychosocial, behavioral, and psychophysiological factors associated with the initiation, exacerbation, and/or maintenance of the arrhythmia.

As mentioned earlier, both anxiety and depression have been shown to affect cardiac rate and rhythm and may occur secondary to the arrhythmia, contributing to its exacerbation. Therefore, an assessment of these psychological factors often provides useful information. If anxiety or depression is known to have existed for some period, effective treatment of the arrhythmia may require treating the underlying psychological disorder. While a comprehensive behavioral assessment is beyond the scope of most cardiological practices, an understanding of the principles involved in such an evaluation should help doctors identify individuals with these psychological disorders.

The assessment of both anxiety and depression requires a multilevel approach. In particular, an adequate assessment should include data derived from three broad areas: self-report, behavioral observation, and physiological assessment.

At the cornerstone of all psychological evaluation is the patient's report. Although some patients with psychological disorders are either unaware of or unable to articulate the nature of their difficulties, most patients report psychological symptoms. Therefore, a description of these symptoms provides a useful starting point for the evaluation. A primary tool in this endeavor is the clinical interview. The mental status examination may provide an initial screening for gross indications of psychopathology. Generally, however, a more extensive interview is necessary for information pertaining to anxiety or depression. An initial outline of problem areas identified by the patient will provide a structure for more detailed analysis. The evaluator should determine whether the reported problems fit a pattern consistent with that seen in anxiety or depression. The *Diagnostic and Statistical Manual of Mental Disorders* (American Psychiatric Association, 1980) provides good descriptions of symptoms associated with these disorders. While fitting the pattern of symptoms to a particular disorder is a necessary process, a conceptual interpretation of how the individual's presenting problems are integrated is often more useful clinically.

Several issues appear important in determining how symptoms of depression or anxiety relate to cardiac arrhythmias. In particular, the patient's perception of his medical disorder may lead to a variety of different behavioral adjustments. The patient who is preoccupied with the negative health consequences of the diagnosis of arrhythmia may likely become depressed or anxious, particularly if other cardiovascular risk factors are apparent. For instance, younger persons with a positive family history of early cardiovascular-related morbidity may vigilantly scan for symptoms and then mistakenly attribute these symptoms to an impending MI. Ultimately, this vigilant focusing may lead to increased sympathetic arousal and subsequent amplification of symptoms (Barsky and Klerman, 1983).

Besides the patient's perception of his illness and attributions, style of coping will influence psychological adjustment. There are several aspects of coping style, including dimensions of activity, passivity, denial, minimizing the seriousness of the symptoms, seeking relevant information, requesting support from social and medical systems, learning specific illness-related procedures, setting concrete goals, and rehearsing alternative outcomes (Moos, 1977). Each should be briefly investigated in a given patient.

An analysis of developmental history and social systems is also important. A thorough history will facilitate this aspect of the interview. Information from these areas enables the examiner to determine recurring or structured behavior patterns. Often interviews with family members will help to clarify these patterns. The history should include information regarding earlier experiences of psychological distress, school and occupational history, previous examples of social and familial relationships, and examples of the individual's way of coping with stress and life needs. An assessment of the current social/family system may provide evidence for factors that interact with and possibly exacerbate the reported symptoms. An assessment of the spouse's perception of and response to the disorder is also useful. In addition to these areas, the interviewer should assess in detail the individual's current vocational and home environment, looking for both physical and psychosocial stressors.

Following the interview, additional information may be obtained from psychometric testing, including self-report inventories. These measures are useful in that they provide a structured means of data collection, frequently require only a minimum of professional time to administer, and are relatively cost-efficient. Several good inventories exist for the evaluation of anxiety (Nietzel and Bernstein, 1981) and mood fluctuation in general (MacKay, 1980). In addition to measures of anxiety, it is often useful to identify specific sources of strain within the work and family environments of these patients. Two psychometric tests developed for this purpose are the Work and Family Environment Scales (Moos, 1981; Moos and Moos, 1981). Table 3 provides an overview of the specific areas measured by these scales.

Table 3. Family and Work Environment Scales:
Subscales and Dimension Descriptions.

FAMILY ENVIRONMENT SCALE

Relationship Dimensions

1. Cohesion	the degree of commitment, help, and support family members provide for one another
2. Expressiveness	the extent to which family members are encouraged to act openly and to express their feelings directly
3. Conflict	the amount of openly expressed anger, aggression, and conflict among family members

Personal Growth Dimensions

4. Independence	the extent to which family members are assertive, are self-sufficient, and make their own decisions
5. Achievement Orientation	the extent to which activities (such as school and work) are cast into an achievement-oriented or competitive framework
6. Intellectual-Cultural Orientation	the degree of interest in political, social, intellectual, and cultural activities
7. Active-Recreational Orientation	the extent of participation in social and recreational activities

Table 3. Family and Work Environment Scales:
Subscales and Dimension Descriptions, Cont'd.

8. Moral-Religious Emphasis	the degree of emphasis on ethical and religious issues and values

System Maintenance Dimensions

9. Organization	the degree of importance of clear organization and structure in planning family activities and responsibilities
10. Control	the extent to which set rules and procedures are used to run family life

WORK ENVIRONMENT SCALE

Relationship Dimensions

1. Involvement	the extent to which employees are concerned about and committed to their jobs
2. Peer Cohesion	the extent to which employees are friendly and supportive of one another
3. Supervisor Support	the extent to which management is supportive of employees and encourages employees to be supportive of one another

Personal Growth Dimensions

4. Autonomy	the extent to which employees are encouraged to be self-sufficient and to make their own decisions
5. Task Orientation	the degree of emphasis on good planning, efficiency, and getting the job done
6. Work Pressure	the degree to which the press of work and time urgency dominate the job milieu

System Maintenance and System Change Dimensions

7. Clarity	the extent to which employees know what to expect in their daily routine and how explicitly rules and policies are communicated
8. Control	the extent to which management uses rules and pressures to keep employees under control
9. Innovation	the degree of emphasis on variety, change, and new approaches
10. Physical Comfort	the extent to which the physical surroundings contribute to a pleasant work environment

Commonly used inventories for the assessment of depression include the Beck Depression Inventory, the Lubin Depression Adjective Checklist, and the Zung Self-Rating Depression Scale (Rehm, 1981). These scales, which provide quantifiable indicators of affective disorders, allow the clinician to compare the patient to depressed populations. In addition, the Minnesota Multiphasic Personality Inventory (MMPI) enables one to assess overall psychological disturbance, particularly relevant to anxiety, depression, and somatization (Dahlstrom, Welsh, and Dahlstrom, 1975).

Frequently decisions must be made regarding the suitability of a particular patient for a biobehavioral approach. While there are no empirically derived decision rules to follow, this decision can often be facilitated by obtaining measures of illness behavior (Pilowsky and Spence, 1976), alexithymia (Apfel and Sifneos, 1979; Lesser, 1981), and self-control behaviors (Rosenbaum, 1980). Through the use of the Illness Behavior Questionnaire, one can obtain information on such factors as disease conviction, hypochrondriasis, and psychological versus somatic perception of illness. While developed with chronic pain patients, the scale appears to be useful with several types of patients with chronic illness. The Shalling-Sifneos Personality Scale provides a simple index of certain aspects of alexithymia (marked problems in verbal expression of emotions). Such patients have been found, anecdotally, to respond poorly to more traditional psychotherapeutic approaches and also to display problems with certain aspects of stress management (for example, identifying sources and signs or reactions to stressors). The Self-Control Schedule measures reported use of self-control strategies in daily living. Since biobehavioral approaches include a focus on self-management and self-control, patients who tend to utilize self-control strategies (use of cognition to control emotional and physiological responses, application of problem-solving strategies, ability to delay gratification) may be more responsive to such approaches.

Direct observation of patients' behavior constitutes the second broad area of evaluation. While formal techniques are available for assessing the occurrence of depression and anxiety through role play or naturalistic observation, the most useful clinical approach is through the observation of the patient's behavior during the interview. Of particular importance is the identification of inadequate interpersonal skills that may contribute to the clinical manifestations of these disorders. A more detailed description of direct observational procedures in clinical practice can be found in Ciminero, Calhoun, and Adams (1977).

The final area of biobehavioral assessment is the psychophysiological analysis. The purpose of this component is to relate specific psychosocial factors to physiological reactivity in a particular patient. In addition to evaluating general autonomic responsivity, the clinician should assess the specific role of various stressors in exacerbating the cardiac arrhythmia. This type of assessment is also frequently a component in the assessment of anxiety. Specific clinical procedures for such an assessment are discussed in Kallman and Feuerstein (1977, in press) and Ray and Raczynski (1981). Perhaps more useful than the laboratory analysis of psychophysiological response patterns for patients with arrhythmia is the use of ambulatory ECG monitoring in the natural environment.

Since the early ambulatory recordings of Holter, considerable technological advances have been made in ambulatory ECG monitoring, so that there is now a relatively efficient methodology for twenty-four-hour ambulatory recording of patients. Medical centers and smaller hospitals alike utilize ambulatory ECG monitoring to evaluate (1) symptoms suggesting arrhythmia or myocardial ischemia (for example, dyspnea, palpitations, syncope, chest pain, or dizziness), (2) documented changes in ECG in response to a variety of therapeutic modalities in individual patients, (3) individual patients' ECG responses to such environmental factors as return to occupational or recreational activities (physical rehabilitation) after MI or cardiac surgery, and (4) clinical syndromes (such as post-MI, cardiomyopathy, mitral valve prolapse, and chronic hemodialysis) and environmental situations where arrhythmias may increase the risk of sudden cardiac death. Although activity-related arrhythmias may be evaluated by means of exercise stress testing, symptoms assumed to be associated with rest or emotional factors may be advantageously assessed by ambulatory monitoring. With ambulatory monitoring the patient can intentionally interact with suspected stressors in the natural environment as a challenge while such interactions are carefully identified on tape along with multiple ECG tracings. An alternative to such a challenge test is the use of ECG monitoring over days while the patient goes about his or her typical activities until a symptom and/or specific stressful encounter or situation ensues, at which time an event marker is used to indicate onset and termination of the event. This latter approach appears to be a more valid representation of the actual *in vivo* psychophysiological process. There are no systematic studies, however, comparing the differential utility of the two strategies (challenge versus natural evolution). The use of ambulatory monitoring also proves useful in patients who are unaware that emotional factors may exacerbate their problems. Such a technique with specific graphic feedback of the time-locked association of stressor-arrhythmia tends to facilitate an appreciation of the link—an important step in a biobehavioral treatment program.

While there are advantages to a dynamic ambulatory ECG analysis of select patients with arrhythmia, there are limitations with certain uses of the method. For example, forty-eight-hour ambulatory ECG recordings in a normal population (sixteen to sixty-five years) revealed that 12 percent of the subjects had complex ventricular ectopy and a wide range of rhythm disturbances (Clarke and others, 1976). Twenty-four-hour ECG recordings on men and women (mean age forty-nine years) with no documentable cardiac disease indicated that 46 percent had at least one ventricular premature complex, while 20 percent had more than ten, and 5 percent had more than one hundred per hour (Kostis and others, 1979). In a series of 518 patients with and without cardiac disease, Levine and associates (1978) reported that no symptom or symptom complex correlated closely with any specific arrhythmia. Fifty-one percent of all arrhythmias, including major arrhythmias, were asymptomatic. Of the 47 percent reporting symptoms, 13 percent had an associated arrhythmia, while 34 percent displayed normal ECG at time of symptom. More specifically, only 36 percent of patients with palpitations, 30 percent with syncope or near syncope, 20 percent with chest pain, 17 percent with dyspnea, and 15 percent with dizziness demonstrated a co-occurrence of arrhythmia and diary notation of symptoms. While these data suggest only limited association between symptom and arrhythmia, they do not limit the applicability of ambulatory ECG monitoring for detecting the role of naturally occurring stressors on arrhythmias in select patients. Indeed, these findings caution us about the assumption that such symptoms have a consistent cardiac origin. Clearly, there is no justifiable a priori basis for assuming that each cardiac-like symptom reported reflects a cardiovascular event. In fact, those patients for whom there is no link between symptom and cardiopathology, as measured by an adequate trial of ambulatory monitoring, may represent a clearly different group from those in whom an association is observed, and, as such, might require a different treatment approach (for example, treatment for depression).

When depression is assumed to play a role in the exacerbation and/or maintenance of the disorder, the clinician may consider conducting a Dexamethasone Suppression Test (DST) to provide a biological marker of the depression. The DST is a simple procedure and appears justified when a clear diagnosis of depression may not otherwise be easily established. Cortisol levels during the DST provide an indirect index of neuroendocrine function (hypothalamic-pituitary axis), empirically demonstrated to differ in endogenously depressed individuals. The DST possesses a relatively high degree of specificity, in that 96 percent of nondepressed patients display a normal suppression of cortisol for a twenty-four-hour period following ingestion of oral dexamethasone. The DST also shows a reasonable degree of sensitivity, with approximately 45 percent (range 24–100 percent) of depressed patients displaying abnormal results (Carroll, 1982). Additional findings of interest include normalization of DST with recovery from depression and gradual improvement of DST with treatment, often somewhat prior to apparent clinical recovery. While the test is far from ideal, it can provide an additional piece of information that may assist in identifying biobehavioral factors contributing to the disorder.

An additional area of importance in a comprehensive biobehavioral assessment is the evaluation of health risk behaviors and associated computation of cardiovascular risk ratios. Several patients with various arrhythmias will display health habits that place them at greater risk for subsequent cardiovascular disease. Certain lifestyle factors—such as overeating, improper nutrition, smoking, and inactivity—are often seen in the arrhythmic patient. While a careful interview that incorporates a behavior-analytic model will provide a fairly good picture of the health risk factors, the use of a systematic questionnaire—coupled with measurement of levels of fitness, systemic blood pressure, and fractionated cholesterol—often provides the information for a *health risk appraisal* or *health risk profile*. The health risk appraisal is an approach that incorporates health-related behaviors, personal characteristics, and physiological parameters in order to estimate an individual's risk of cardiovascular morbidity and mortality. Through comparison with morbidity, mortality, and other epidemiological data, risk ratios are computed and typically presented in a form suggesting that modification in certain behaviors contributing to the risk may result in a reduction in subsequent risk. An example of a page from one of the more thoughtful health risk appraisals is shown in Figure 2.

The health risk appraisal approach, while still in its infancy clinically, appears promising when combined with a health promotion protocol (Rodnick, 1982). In a review of this approach, Wagner and associates (1982) point to a number of assets and problems. Assets include (1) provision of a rationale and teaching aid in discussions on health and behavior; (2) reliance on self-administered questionnaires, simple physiological measurement, and computer-assisted calculations, resulting in an efficient and relatively inexpensive device; (3) scientific appearance and foundation, with emphasis on numbers and computer-generated reports; and (4) consistency with current zeitgeist regarding lifestyle and health. Limitations include (1) emphasis on self-report; (2) continuing controversy among epidemiologists over the predictive utility of risk ratios and the fact that some instruments attempt to predict events where little or no data exist to support such predictions; (3) questionable applicability for younger patients (under thirty-five years

Figure 2. Example of a Health Risk Appraisal Report.

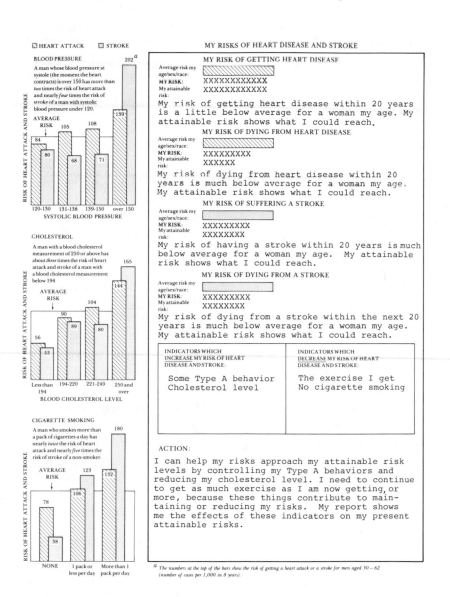

of age), since most of the risk factors are based on studies of
older individuals; and (4) applicability confinement to white,
middle-class individuals, because of limited data on minority
individuals. In addition, to understand this type of analysis, participants generally need a higher than average educational background.

Notwithstanding the limitations of health risk appraisals,
data are available suggesting moderate effects of the health risk
appraisal on reduction of physiological risk variables (such as
high blood pressure and cholesterol) and some change in such
risk behaviors as cigarette smoking and lack of exercise (Milsum, 1980; Rodnick, 1982). From a clinical perspective, we
have found that a careful review of the results of a health risk
appraisal by practitioner and patient provides a structured
springboard for systematic efforts at cardiovascular risk reduction.

The following case provides a brief example of an evaluation and conceptualization of a patient with arrhythmia and
multiple somatic complaints referred to our clinic.

R. L. was a thirty-three-year-old married male, with
young children two and four years old, referred by GI Medicine
to the Pain and Stress Management Laboratory with diagnoses
of irritable bowel syndrome and cardiac arrhythmia. Medical
chart review documents a long history of epigastric and retro-
sternal discomfort, as well as anxiety. Upper GI series have
shown a hiatal hernia with gastroesphogeal reflux. Gallbladder
studies have been negative. A twenty-four-hour Holter monitor
showed evidence of proxysmal atrial tachycardia in one short
burst that was unaccompanied by significant symptoms. R. L.'s
concern over cardiac problems developed recently, while the GI
complaints are longstanding. It is relevant to note that the patient's father died of a myocardial infarction at forty-three
years. There is also a family history of hypertension and mitral
valve prolapse. When the patient was referred, he was taking
Xanax (.5 mg three times a day), Deseryl (50 mg at night), Lopressor (25 mg twice a day), Zantac (140 mg twice a day), and
Combid (one tablet twice a day). At this time R. L. does not

smoke and drinks alcohol twice a month, though prior to the past year he had smoked one to one and a half packs a day and had drunk seven or eight alcoholic drinks a night.

The patient described a ten-year history of problems with painful abdominal bloating and burning sensations of discomfort. He believed that his symptoms had become progressively severe. His last severe episode had included chest pressure, intense squeezing pain, racing heartbeat, light-headedness, and a sense of suffocating and panic. He also described problems with cramping, diarrhea, and constipation. Although he believed that his problems had some undiagnosed physical basis, he also was willing to consider that stress at work, related to problems with co-workers, sometimes aggravated his symptoms. R. L. had his physician's agreement in taking a medical leave of absence from work and had been out of work two months when first seen.

Psychological testing offered no evidence of severe psychopathology. However, R. L. seemed to be preoccupied with somatic concerns and mildly depressed. He may use denial to cope with psychological difficulties. Further testing (Illness Behavior Questionnaire) revealed that R. L. ruminates about his symptoms, is fearful of exacerbations of his illness, and is made irritable by his illness. He reported using self-control behaviors to deal with problems in daily living (Self-Control Scale). He felt that his family environment was nonproblematic (Family Environment Scale); however, he viewed his work situation as having low peer cohesion and reported a low personal investment in his work (Work Environment Scale). On the McGill Pain Questionnaire, R. L. described his pain as "shooting, stabbing, exhausting, suffocating"—suggesting both sensory and affective components to his pain. He displayed no pain behavior during the interview.

Three major target areas were identified: (1) excessive dysfunctional autonomic arousal, (2) maladaptive cognitions regarding health status and symptoms, and (3) avoidant behaviors. Excessive autonomic activity was evidenced by increased heart rate, bloating, gastroesophageal reflux, acidity, diarrhea, constipation, light-headedness, and panic. The maladaptive cognitions regarding his health were directed at (1) feelings of helplessness when symptoms occur (for example, "When these symptoms occur, I can't perform my job duties," "I just can't handle these feelings in my stomach and chest"), (2) catastrophic expectations when symptoms occur ("I might pass out, aspirate on my vomit, and strangulate while unconscious"), and (3) negative attitudes regarding diagnosis and health care ("The diagnoses I received are wastebasket terms, and I don't believe it when they tell me there is nothing seriously wrong with me"). Avoidant behaviors included postponing return to work, avoidance of any exercise or physical activity, and avoidance of social activities with friends.

The specific treatment goals were (1) decreased symptoms, (2) resumption of work and of physical and social activity, and (3) reduced dependence on medication (Xanax, Deseryl, and Lopressor). Treatment strategies directed at these goals focused on decreasing autonomic arousal and modifying maladaptive cognitions.

Review of Treatment Literature

The various treatments reported in the literature include heart rate biofeedback, relaxation therapy, meditation, hypnosis, and psychotherapy. Two basic treatment rationales provide the foundation for the use of these interventions. The first is related to relaxation therapy, meditation, and hypnosis. These procedures are assumed to assist in the reduction of high levels of physiological/autonomic arousal and/or reactivity if coupled with some form of systematic desensitization or stress inoculation training. As discussed in an earlier section, the increased arousal may represent a "final common pathway" in the exacerbation and/or triggering of arrhythmic activity. While the literature provides reports on the three procedures indicated above, theoretically any technique directed at reducing autonomic arousal (for instance, aerobics) could result in a reduction in arrhythmic activity. Indeed, reduction of autonomic arousal may have been the mechanism accounting for reductions in ventricular arrhythmias following group psychotherapy (Gruen, 1975).

The second major treatment reported in the literature is

biofeedback, thought to represent a more specific and direct approach to arrhythmias than the relaxation-based approaches. In a biofeedback treatment paradigm for arrhythmia, the patient's heart rate or cardiac conduction is monitored. This cardiac activity is fed back to the patient in the form of a digital display, a light, or a tone indicating the status of the patient's heart rate or conduction. The patient is instructed to use this information to develop various cognitive and/or physiological strategies (for example, to visualize heart rhythm stabilizing/slowing) to produce specific cardiac responses. As the responses are achieved, the patient receives the self-reward of success and continues to achieve greater control over the target response. The desired outcome of this type of training is the self-regulation of a cardiac response in absence of feedback in the patient's natural environment. Although cardiac biofeedback was represented by a substantial number of reports in the literature prior to 1980, it has not been readily adopted in clinical practice—possibly because of the complexity of the procedure with arrhythmias, the length of time required for a desired effect, and the lack of evidence for its superiority over other approaches. Few reports of its use have been published since 1980.

The following literature review is organized according to specific classes of arrhythmias.

Single Ectopic Beats. Pickering and Miller (1977) report findings from two well-documented cases. The first patient was a fourteen-year-old boy with a two-and-a-half-year history of premature ventricular contractions (PVCs). Therapeutic trials of various antiarrhythmic medications had been unsuccessful. During thirty sessions over six months, the patient learned to maintain a normal sinus rhythm. Feedback consisted of an ECG displayed on an oscilloscope. Occasional trials without feedback were introduced to test his ability to detect PVCs. The ability to identify changes in heart rhythm was never consistent, and he was unable to suppress the PVCs over nine sessions. Following the tenth session, he obtained some control; and during the subsequent nine sessions, the amount of time in normal sinus rhythm increased from 5.2 to 32.7 percent. This patient, however, was unable to maintain normal sinus rhythm without feedback. The second case was a thirty-five-year-old male with a one-year history of PVCs. The PVCs primarily occurred sporadically, although during occasional symptomatic attacks each normal beat was followed by a PVC, resulting in a bigeminal (coupling of the pulse) rhythm. Training sessions were carried out on two separate occasions, five months apart. Training occurred for four consecutive days, with four training sessions per day. The goal of training was increased heart rate. Mode of feedback was a meter display of the cardiotachograph output. During the initial sixteen sessions, the patient learned to raise his heart rate by 20 to 25 beats per minute (BPM) for short periods of time. This increase was associated with a suppression of the bigeminal rhythm. During the subsequent five months, the patient practiced heart rate acceleration, using a cardiac monitor at home. When he was reevaluated in the laboratory, he was able to increase his rate by 20 to 40 BPM with or without feedback and to suppress the bigeminal rhythm approximately 50 percent of the time. With feedback he could modify his heart rate to any given level between 70 and 110 BPM. Toward the end of the second training phase, which followed five months of practice at home, he was able to suppress his PVCs 100 percent of the time. While both cases suggest the potential utility of biofeedback in the management of cardiac arrhythmias, Pickering and Miller indicate that sustained therapuetic benefit was not determined.

Pickering and Gorham (1975) studied a thirty-one-year-old woman with an eight-year history of PVCs, parasystolic in rhythm (at least one ectopic focus fires at a regular and uninterrupted rate in addition to the normal pacemaker), with a frequency of 0 to 15 per minute. The patient was trained to accelerate and decelerate heart rate during sixteen one-hour sessions. Feedback of PVCs was provided by a heart rate meter. During the first six sessions, she was able to increase her heart rate approximately 4.2 BPM. During the final session, she could raise her heart rate by 25 BPM with or without feedback. As the patient learned to increase her heart rate, the threshold for arrhythmias shifted from 79 BPM to 94 BPM. She was much less successful at slowing her heart rate, achieving decreases of only 1 or 2 BPM. No follow-up was reported.

Engel and Bleecker (1974) investigated the effects of heart rate feedback in a twenty-seven-year-old woman diagnosed as having Marfan's syndrome an inherited disease with abnormalities of the skeletal system, eyes, and the cardiovascular system—and a seven-year history of progressive heart failure, which had not been responsive to medical treatment. The patient experienced up to 20 PVCs per minute during two days of baseline measurements. The patient was taught to lower heart rate for four days. She averaged 15 PVCs per minute during the pretraining baseline recording. There was an immediate decrease to 5 PVCs per minute at the onset of training. It is difficult to explain this reduction in arrhythmic activity on the basis of heart rate training, since it occurred before she learned heart rate control. During the fourteen days of heart rate training, her average frequency of PVCs dropped from 5 to almost 0 per minute. Nine months after training, several ten-hour ECG recordings were collected that demonstrated the absence of PVCs. At the follow-up visit, the patient was reported to be working steadily and taking no antiarrhythmic medication.

The use of feedback techniques for single ectopic heartbeats was further demonstrated by Weiss and Engel (1971) in a study of eight patients. The subject sample included two females and six males, who ranged in age from thirty-six to seventy-seven years. These patients were hospitalized during the course of the experiment and had up to three eighty-minute heart rate feedback training sessions daily. Visual feedback consisted of binary heart rate information and a meter that indicated the amount of time the patient was demonstrating control. Heart rate increase and decrease were taught. The patients had approximately ten sessions of training in each of these conditions and were subsequently trained to maintain heart rate within a defined range. During this training feedback availability was progressively limited, in order to "wean" the subjects from feedback. All eight subjects learned some degree of heart rate control. Five were able to control the frequency of PVCs in the laboratory, and four subjects showed decreased PVCs at a follow-up, which in certain cases occurred twenty-one months after training.

There are two reports of nonbiofeedback interventions

for the treatment of patients with single ectopic beats. Collison (1970) reports the use of hypnosis with a sixteen-year-old boy who had a four-year history of frequent ventricular ectopic beats. The subject readily entered a deep trance and was given suggestions of increased relaxation and coping abilities. The number and length of sessions are unspecified. The patient reportedly experienced complete relief and was asymptomatic at a three-year follow-up. Unfortunately, no data on specific ECG changes are provided.

An additional study suggests that Benson's relaxation response may be effective in decreasing the occurrence of PVCs. Benson, Alexander, and Feldman (1975) taught eleven patients —two females and nine males ranging in age from forty-eight to seventy years—the relaxation technique. All the subjects had a diagnosis of ischemic heart disease of at least one-year duration and documented PVCs for which none of the subjects was taking medication. They had one treatment session during which they were taught the relaxation response and instructed to practice the technique for ten to twenty minutes twice a day for one month. The frequency of PVCs was monitored before training and after the month's practice. Reduced PVC frequency was documented in eight of the eleven patients. The average PVCs for all subjects dropped from 151.5 to 131.7 per hour, or from 2.5 to 2.2 per minute. Although this average decrease of .3 PVCs per minute is small, the decrease in three of these patients was over 85 percent. During sleep the average rate of PVCs per hour in these subjects decreased from 125.5 to 87.9.

Multiple Consecutive Ectopic Beats. Scott and associates (1973) report data from two single-subject experiments. One subject was a forty-six-year-old male who had a ten-year history of chronic tachycardia (type unspecified). After two baseline recording sessions, he was trained to decrease heart rate for twenty-two sessions (forty minutes in length with twenty minutes of feedback). During the first thirteen sessions, a meter showing the amount of time the patient was able to decrease his heart rate below a criterion level was used for feedback. For the next nine sessions, the performance criterion was continuously reset in the desired direction to shape the patient's heart rate change. During the last two sessions, the patient was reinforced for his attempts to return his heart rate to the preexperimental baseline level. The constant criterion procedure produced very little change in the patient's heart rate; however, the shaping procedures led to a considerable decrease in heart rate. The patient's preexperimental heart rate averaged 80 BPM; during the last six trials of the shaping procedure, his heart rate averaged 72 BPM. When the patient was instructed to return his heart rate to baseline, it stabilized at 77 BPM. Following training, the patient experienced less anxiety, returned to work, and spontaneously decreased his dosage of a minor tranquilizer. The second subject was a fifty-year-old man who had a twenty-six-year history of anxiety neurosis, including tachycardia (type unspecified). After two baseline recording sessions, this patient was trained to decrease his heart rate during nineteen sessions (forty minutes in length with twenty minutes of feedback), using the shaping procedure. He was then instructed for eight trials to return his heart rate to baseline levels. His average baseline heart rate of 96 BPM dropped 14 BPM after nineteen shaping trials. During the last eight trials, when the patient was retrained to his preexperimental baseline, his heart rate stabilized at 78 BPM. The patient reported that he felt stronger and less anxious and that he was able to perform more household chores without tiring rapidly.

Blanchard and Abel (1976) report a single-subject experiment in which a thirty-year-old woman with a sixteen-year history of episodic tachycardia (type unspecified) received thirty-three sessions of heart rate biofeedback training (twenty minutes of feedback per session). She also participated in group psychotherapy and was stabilized on Dilantin (100 mg per day for brief seizure-like attacks) during the course of the study. Preceding the initiation of biofeedback treatment, she had discovered that her episodes of tachycardia were elicited by specific stressful stimuli. She successfully learned to decrease her heart rate an average of 5 BPM with and without visual heart rate feedback. She was also able to maintain her heart rate decrease in the presence of new stressful stimuli. The patient reported that her episodes of tachycardia had virtually disappeared by the end of the thirty-three training sessions.

Engel and Bleecker (1974) report data from single-subject

experiments with three patients who had various supraventricular tachycardias. The first patient was a forty-one-year-old man with an eight-year history of constant paroxysmal atrial tachycardia and a heart rate that averaged between 130 and 140 BPM. Treatment with medications had been ineffective. During twenty-five half-hour sessions, the patient was taught to slow his heart rate. For the first seventeen sessions, feedback was a display of his electrocardiogram on a calibrated oscilloscope. For the final eight sessions, the patient trained with binary heart rate feedback. The patient was able to slow his heart rate somewhat with the oscilloscope feedback, but he was more effective at regulating his heart rate with binary feedback. By the seventeenth session, he had established a new resting heart rate 15 BPM below his pretreatment level. During the subsequent five months, the patient's heart rate ranged from 60 to 75 BPM, and his symptoms of congestive heart failure disappeared.

Engel and Bleecker report a second patient with a sinus tachycardia. This patient was a fifty-three-year-old woman with an average heart rate of 106 BPM who had not been observed to have a heart rate below 80 BPM for the four years prior to the study. She was trained to decrease her heart rate over twenty-one sessions. For the first eleven sessions, she received constant visual binary heart rate feedback. For the final nine sessions (forty-eight minutes in length), the percentage of time that feedback was available was progressively reduced to help her become less dependent on visual feedback to control her heart rate. She was equally successful in lowering her heart rate with and without feedback. Her pulse dropped from 86 BPM at the start of the study to 68 BPM in later sessions. Along with this change, her blood pressure decreased from 140/80 mg Hg to 115/75 mm Hg.

The third case was a thirty-six-year-old woman with a two-year history of one episode of paroxysmal atrial tachycardia (PAT) per month and occasional periods of sinus tachycardia. This patient was trained to slow her heart rate for twenty seventeen-minute sessions and to increase her heart rate during an additional ten sessions. During eight sessions of differential heart rate training, she was instructed to raise and then lower her heart rate. Although this patient was able to slow her heart rate only minimally, she was able to increase it consistently by 7 to 20 BPM. Surprisingly, she reported less anxiety when she had a faster heart rate. At a six-month follow-up, she reported only one episode of tachycardia, which she was able to control voluntarily.

Bleecker and Engel (1973a) employed a similar experimental procedure with three women and three men who had chronic atrial fibrillation. They ranged in age from twenty-eight to sixty-two years and had had symptoms for two to twenty years. All of them had rheumatic heart disease, which had been stabilized with digitalis for at least three months. They were taught to increase their ventricular rate (VR) for ten sessions, to slow it for ten sessions, and alternately to speed and slow it for another ten sessions. All biofeedback sessions were seventeen minutes long, with continuous visual binary feedback of ventricular rate. Two subjects were consistently able to increase their rate, two were better at slowing their rate, and the remaining two subjects were best at differentially increasing and slowing their ventricular rates. On the average, subjects learned to increase VR by 9.5 BPM and to slow it by 3.5 BPM. All subjects were able differentially to increase and slow their ventricular contraction rate during the alternation phase of training. All subjects significantly modified the frequency distributions of their R-R intervals. Two subjects received extensive training to decrease ventricular rate variability. While both were able to reduce this variability with feedback, neither subject showed any reduction of VR variability in the absence of feedback. This study demonstrates that patients with chronic atrial fibrillation prescribed digitalis can learn to control ventricular rate.

Although biofeedback is the most frequently reported psychological technique for the treatment of tachycardia, meditation, psychotherapy, and hypnosis have also been used. Lown and colleagues (1976) studied meditation as a treatment in a thirty-nine year-old man with two episodes of ventricular fibrillation related to "nervous activity." The patient was taught a transcendental meditation–like procedure and practiced this meditation twice daily while viewing his ECG on an oscilloscope.

While meditating, the patient attempted to suppress his PVCs. After one week, he was able to reduce their frequency from 11 per minute to 3 per minute. Nine months later he had no PVCs. The effect of meditation, however, was confounded by the feedback procedure, a regular exercise program, verbalization of dreams, and antiarrhythmic drugs.

Collison (1970) describes the use of hypnosis for the treatment of various tachycardias. A thirty-six-year-old man with a ten-year history of paroxysmal ventricular tachycardia, which was unsuccessfully treated with quinidine and sedatives, was given relaxing hypnotic suggestions. He was seen for hypnotherapy daily for an unspecified length of time as an inpatient, and then weekly and biweekly for a total of six months. After treatment the tachycardia occurred only sporadically, and at three-year follow-up the patient reported only mild recurrences of the symptom. Collison also used hypnosis with three women (twenty-two to thirty-five years old) who suffered from paroxysmal atrial tachycardia (PAT). These patients received relaxation suggestions designed to help them cope with various life situations. The number and length of sessions are unspecified. One patient experienced immediate relief, a second patient showed a decrease in the frequency of episodes of PAT from several weekly to one every ten to twelve weeks, and the third patient reported no change in symptoms. The long-term effects of this procedure are not reported.

Rahe and Christ (1966) used psychotherapy and family therapy to treat an eleven-year-old boy who developed paroxysmal ventricular tachycardia. The parents monitored their son's pulse and observed his emotional state. This monitoring reportedly helped them understand the psychological factors influencing the tachycardia. At the same time, the patient was seen weekly for individual play therapy, the patient's mother was seen for weekly individual psychotherapy, and the parents had monthly couples-therapy sessions. After one year of treatment in conjunction with antiarrhythmic drugs, improvement was noted in the patient's levels of enjoyment and relaxation and in the parents' ability to interact with their son with confidence and firmness. Other than one stress-related episode of tachycardia, the patient was reported to have remained in good health.

Gruen (1975) compared a group of recent myocardial infarction (MI) patients ($N = 33$) who were seen for thirty-minute daily psychotherapy sessions with a similar group of patients ($N = 35$) who were not seen in therapy. The occurrence of arrhythmias recorded during two daily five-minute samples (seven to eleven days post-MI) was tabulated for both groups of patients. It was found that 15 percent of the treated patients, as compared to 29 percent of the controls, experienced ventricular arrhythmias and that 5 percent of the treated patients and 23 percent of the controls had supraventricular arrhythmias. This decrease in incidence of arrhythmias in the treatment group—along with decreases in reported weakness and depression, fewer days of intensive care, and less anxiety when measured at four-month follow-up—supports the use of psychotherapy during recovery from an MI. Because of the sporadic and limited collection of ECG data, definitive conclusions regarding the impact of psychotherapy on cardiac pathology in this group must await replication incorporating appropriate cardiovascular measures.

Disturbance of Impulse Conduction and Combined Impulse Formation and Conduction. Engel and Bleecker (1974) studied three patients with third-degree heart block treated with biofeedback training to speed ventricular rate. None of the patients was able consistently to increase his ventricular rate. Bleecker and Engel (1973b) also used biofeedback to assist a twenty-nine-year-old woman with a ten-year history of Wolff-Parkinson-White (WPW) syndrome. She was taught to lower heart rate (twenty-six sessions), raise heart rate (fifteen sessions), and alternately increase and slow heart rate (twenty-one sessions). She was then taught to increase the frequency of WPW conduction and the frequency of normal conduction. For seventeen minutes of each session, she received binary feedback, which was presented to her visually during heart rate training and aurally during heart rhythm training. At the end of this treatment, she could decrease her heart rate 3.4 BPM, increase her heart rate 2.5 BPM, and successfully change from increased to decreased heart rate or vice versa during twenty of twenty-one test sessions. She was also able to increase the proportion of normally conducted beats by 13 percent with and without feedback. Follow-up after ten weeks showed that she could continue to control her cardiac conduction.

Clinical Implications. Definitive conclusions regarding the efficacy of biofeedback, relaxation, meditation, hypnosis, and psychotherapy with cardiac arrhythmias cannot be made. The clinical studies reported are limited by the use of multiple interventions, which prevent the identification of the active treatment components. Many reports do not describe the treatment setting (inpatient or outpatient); the length of treatment sessions and duration of treatment; the use of concurrent medication, including antiarrhythmic agents; or the specific type of arrhythmia. Many of the case reports also do not provide sufficient information to allow replication. The most serious clinical limitation is the lack of clinical outcome data, which must include a description of generalization of treatment effects to the patient's home environment. Given these limitations, only tentative conclusions can be drawn.

Heart rate control achieved through heart rate feedback training results in the elimination or reduction in the frequency of PVCs in approximately 50 percent of the cases. The training procedure that appears to be most effective is one including training sessions in heart rate deceleration, acceleration, and combined deceleration and acceleration, as well as sessions that train the patient to maintain his heart rate within a fixed range. The use of analogue or continuous visual feedback of the patient's ECG is not as effective as binary (on/off as function of occurrence of interior response) feedback. The effects of hypnotic procedures on ectopic beats are unclear. An anecdotal report suggests remission of arrhythmias in one case at three-year follow-up. However, this conclusion is not supported with ECG data, and further research is clearly needed in this area. Relaxation training for treating PVCs appears to be promising. While the reported efficacy is based on short-term follow-up studies, this technique does appear to be effective in reducing the frequency of PVCs in certain patients. Patient factors associated with positive response have not been delineated. Given its sim-

plicity and low cost, the clinical use of relaxation training warrants serious consideration.

Heart rate biofeedback appears to be useful in the treatment of tachycardia (type unspecified). Specifically, training
in heart rate deceleration seems to assist in the management of
stress-related tachycardia. It also appears that biofeedback training for stress-induced tachycardia may be facilitated by teaching
heart rate regulation in the presence of stressful stimuli. A binary feedback approach to train heart rate deceleration has
been the most common therapeutic strategy. A continuous
visual display of ECG is not as useful. The effects of nonbiofeedback procedures for tachycardia are difficult to evaluate.
Unfortunately, few specific data were provided to describe
changes in the frequency of target problems. These studies do
suggest, however, that the use of hypnosis, self-monitoring of
pulse and emotional level, and psychotherapy may be useful in
the treatment of tachycardia. A more detailed description of
some useful techniques is given in the next section. Biofeedback and other biobehavioral techniques do not appear to be
very useful in the treatment of third-degree heart block. However, increases in normal cardiac conduction and decreases in
heart rate have been reported in one patient with Wolff-Parkinson-White syndrome.

It has been proposed that a possible "final common pathway" for the effects of various biobehavioral techniques is a
general relaxation response with a concomitant reduction in
sympathetic nervous system arousal (Silver and Blanchard,
1978; Stoyva and Budzynski, 1974). This arousal reduction hypothesis is consistent with information on the role of sympathetic activity in the exacerbation of arrhythmias. If reduction
of sympathetic arousal is a clinical goal in the management of
patients with arrhythmia, heart rate biofeedback does not appear to be an efficient approach to achieve this goal. Various
management procedures are available that develop a more enduring set of stress reduction skills, often within a shorter period of time. Reduction of sympathetic arousal should be viewed
as only one of several treatment goals. The patient with arrhythmia may also show significant depression, somatization, and a

pattern of risk behaviors associated with the exacerbation of the arrhythmia; and these disorders also would require clinical attention.

Treatment Protocol

As indicated in earlier sections, a treatment program for arrhythmias, as with any disorder, should follow a complete evaluation from medical and biobehavioral vantage points. Such an evaluation generally suggests a set of clinical procedures directed at identifiable target areas. Essentially, from a biobehavioral perspective, these target problems include anxiety, depression, and cardiovascular risk behaviors. A comprehensive treatment program is directed at the modification of those components present in a given patient.

Anxiety/Stress Management. A variety of treatment options are available for the management of anxiety/stress. These techniques include biofeedback (electromyographic, skin temperature, skin conductance), progressive relaxation training, autogenic training, and aerobic exercise. These techniques are directed primarily at the physiological component of the anxiety or stress response. Systematic desensitization may also prove useful in cases where the arrhythmias appear to be triggered by specific events. When a behavioral component to the anxiety/stress response is observed (for example, avoidance or aggression), and it has been determined that specific behavioral skills (such as assertiveness, communication, or social skills) are lacking, such skills should be targeted for intervention. If a considerable cognitive component appears to be contributing to subjective distress and/or repeated physiological arousal, this area also should be addressed. Such cognitive techniques as developed by Ellis and Abrahams (1978) and Beck (1976) are quite useful, particularly if the level of psychopathology is minimal.

In cases where more than one component of the stress response is apparent, a stress inoculation training approach, as developed by Meichenbaum (1977) and subsequently elaborated on by Meichenbaum and Cameron (1983), provides a useful framework for anxiety/stress management. It is a framework that is conceptually and technically easy to understand and implement for both patient and nonpsychological/psychiatric clinician, and therefore provides a practical model for the management of the anxiety/stress component of the arrhythmic patient's complaints. However, the patient's overall presenting problems may not be as simple as this model is. Therefore, the clinician must obtain a *comprehensive* history in order to determine the basis for the anxiety/stress.

Table 4 specifies the treatment paradigm for stress inoculation training. The program is divided into three general phases: conceptualization, skills acquisition/rehearsal, and application/ follow-through. The interested reader should refer to Meichenbaum and Cameron (1983) for a more detailed review.

Table 4. A Flow Chart of Stress Inoculation Training.

Phase One: Conceptualization

(a) Data collection–integration
- Identify determinants of problem via interview, image-based reconstruction, self-monitoring, and behavioral observation
- Distinguish between performance failure and skill deficit
- Formulate treatment plan—task analysis
- Introduce integrative conceptual model

(b) Assessment skills training
- Train clients to analyze problems independently (for example, to conduct situational analyses and to seek disconfirmatory data)

Phase Two: Skills Acquisition and Rehearsal

(a) Skills training
- Train instrumental coping skills (for example, communication, assertion, problem solving, parenting, study skills)
- Train palliative coping skills as indicated (for example, perspective taking, attention diversion, use of social supports, adaptive affect expression, relaxation)
- Aim to develop an extensive repertoire of coping responses to facilitate flexible responding

(b) Skills Rehearsal
- Promote smooth integration and execution of coping responses via imagery and role play
- Self-instructional training to develop mediators to regulate coping responses

(continued on next page)

Table 4. A Flow Chart of Stress Inoculation Training, Cont'd.

Phase Three: Application and Follow-Through

(a)   Induce application of skills
  • Prepare for application using coping imagery, using early stress cues as signals to cope
  • Role play (a) anticipated stressful situations and (b) client coaching someone with a similar problem
  • "Role-play" attitude may be adopted in real world
  • Exposure to in-session graded stressors
  • Use of graded exposure and other response induction aids to foster *in vivo* responding and build self-efficacy
(b)   Maintenance and generalization
  • Build sense of coping self-efficacy in relation to situations client sees as high risk
  • Develop strategies for recovering from failure and relapse
  • Arrange follow-up reviews

General Guidelines for Training

  • Attend to referral and intake process
  • Consider training peers of clients to conduct treatment. Develop collaborative relationship and project approachability
  • Establish realistic expectations regarding course and outcome of therapy
  • Foster optimism and confidence by structuring incremental success experiences
  • Respond to stalled progress with problem solving versus labeling client resistant
  • Include family members in treatment where this is indicated

---

Reproduced, with permission of the publisher and the authors, from D. Meichenbaum and R. Cameron, "Stress Inoculation Training." In D. Meichenbaum and M. E. Jaemko (Eds.), *Stress Reduction and Prevention* (New York: Plenum, 1983).

Essentially, the conceptualization phase includes collection and integration of data and relates to several of the issues raised in the previous section on evaluation. This phase is also designed to enhance the problem-solving skills of the patient by training the patient to perform a situational analysis. Data are obtained through clinical interview; image-based reconstruction of the various stressors, including focus on self-statements or cognitive appraisals of the events; self-monitoring; and behavioral observation. Once these data are integrated, the clinician then places them in some overall perspective for the patient, in order to explain why and how his response to stress has evolved and is currently being maintained. In the second phase, the goal is to help the patient develop and implement coping responses, such as perspective taking, attention diversion, increasing social support networks, appropriate expression of affect, and learning of relaxation skills. These newly developed coping responses are rehearsed both in the therapy sessions, and in relatively safe situations in the extratherapeutic environment. Self-instructional training (that is, the use of coping self-statements and directions) is also frequently suggested as a means of directing a patient through a stressful situation. The therapist continually monitors the specific thoughts and feelings the patient experiences at each phase of the stress reaction—including preparation for the stressor, confronting the stressor, and critical moments of intense stress—and during periods of reflection regarding the actual handling of the stressful event.

Finally, in the application/follow-though phase, the coping responses are directed at behavior change in real-world situations and at long-term change. During this phase the patient is helped to identify high-risk situations and to deal with failure. As delineated by Meichenbaum and Cameron (1983), this approach includes five common elements: (1) teaching patients the role that cognitions and emotions play in the modulation of the stress response; (2) training in self-monitoring of stress-exacerbating thoughts, images, feelings, and behaviors; (3) training in problem solving; (4) modeling and rehearsing of coping skills; and (5) graded *in vivo* behavioral assignments of increasing difficulty.

Depression. For the short-term management of depression, Beck's cognitive therapy (Beck, 1976) and Lewinsohn's behavioral therapy (Lewinsohn, Sullivan, and Grosscup, 1982) models are useful. Briefly, the rationale for Beck's cognitive therapy is that depression is best conceptualized as a disturbance in cognition. Rather than a primary disturbance of mood, depression is hypothesized as the result of distorted, negatively biased views of self, future, and world; this cognitive distortion influences the affective, motivational, behavioral, and vegetative manifestations of depression. Therefore, the goal of such therapy is to enable the patient to develop a more accurate view of self, future, and world. Techniques such as self-monitoring, activities scheduling, graded task assignments, cognitive rehearsal, role playing, and self-help homework assignments are used to help the patient (1) elicit automatic (maladaptive) thoughts, (2) test automatic thoughts, (3) identify maladaptive underlying assumptions, and (4) analyze the validity of maladaptive assumptions. A detailed description of this approach is available (Beck and others, 1979). We have found the approach particularly useful in patients for whom cognitive distortions appear prominent in the depression.

In cases where the symptoms appear to be the consequence of reduced environmental reinforcement (that is, the patient's interaction with the environment results in limited positive outcomes), a more behavioral approach often proves useful. The rationale underlying this approach is that a low rate of response-contingent reinforcement or increased rates of punishment constitute important antecedents for the occurrence of depression. These environmental consequences result in a reduced quality of environmental interaction, which in turn results in a reduction in social behavior (increased passivity) and the dysphoric feelings central to depression. This model proposes three possibilities for the experience of low rates of positive reinforcement and/or high rates of punishment: (1) availability of reinforcers/punishers in the immediate environment, (2) lack of skills necessary to obtain available positive reinforcers and/or cope with aversive events, and (3) reduction in the strength of a positively reinforcing event and/or increased negative impact of a punishing event. The goal of treatment from this perspective is to increase the patient's rate (quantity and quality) of positively reinforcing interactions with the environment while simultaneously decreasing punishing interactions. The techniques useful to achieve these goals include self-monitoring of unpleasant events and mood, increasing pleasant activities, and a variety of behavioral techniques specific to target problem areas (for example, social skills training). The Lewinsohnian approach provides a useful set of techniques for the patient with considerable illness behavior and associated low activity level, since it facilitates increased interaction with the environment.

The cognitive and behavioral approaches are not incompatible and, in fact, complement each other well in patients whose depression appears to be the result of both cognitive distortion and environmental reinforcement deficits.

Health Risk Reduction/Health Enhancement. As pointed out earlier, certain behaviors are associated with the etiology and/or exacerbation of arrhythmias. Such habits as smoking and coffee ingestion can contribute directly to the short-term exacerbation of arrhythmias, while smoking, inactive lifestyle, diet, and Type A behavior can contribute to longer-term development of arrhythmias and additional cardiovascular disease, placing the arrhythmic patient at greater risk. Consequently, efforts directed at modifying these behaviors represent good clinical practice.

There are a number of approaches useful in the modification of health habits. A review of such approaches is beyond the focus of this chapter, and some are discussed in other chapters in this volume. In general, however, the literature indicates that no one particular approach is superior to any others at present. Also, the literature and clinical experience indicate that short-term reduction or elimination of a specific health risk behavior is more easily achieved than long-term maintenance of change (Zifferblatt and Wilbur, 1977). This is particularly the case with smoking and dieting (Brownell, 1982), although similar findings have been reported for activity/exercise (Martin and Dubbert, 1982). Recently efforts have been made to develop approaches to facilitate long-term change in health behavior. This work suggests that such factors as social support and incentive systems assist in achieving these goals (Davidson and Davidson, 1980).

Health promotion programs have recently been developed at work sites (Fielding, 1982). Some of these programs provide continuous monitoring and follow-up, along with considerable social support and incentive programs assisting in longer-term compliance. Such substantial support can be approximated only rarely in a clinical setting. Therefore, when patients present with risk factors potentially contributing to their arrhythmias, we recommend that they enroll in work site or other community group programs after obtaining clearance from their primary physicians or cardiologists. As discussed earlier, the health risk appraisal provides a useful tool to educate the patient about the role of risk factors and often facilitates the transition from awareness of a risk factor to participation in a health risk reduction program, particularly if the health risk report is carefully reviewed with the patient.

While the treatment of the patient with arrhythmia varies as a function of the pattern of presenting problems, the following case provides an example of treatment from a biobehavioral perspective.

R. L. (whose case was described in the section on "Evaluation of the Patient with Arrhythmias") was seen in outpatient treatment for sixteen one-hour weekly sessions over a six-month period. Treatment goals were specified and jointly agreed upon to include (1) decrease in symptoms, (2) resumption of work and of physical and social activities, and (3) decreased use of medication. The treatment procedure used to reduce the autonomically mediated symptoms included progressive muscle relaxation training followed by skin conductance biofeedback-assisted relaxation, relaxation-deepening techniques, and self-hypnosis. These techniques were the major focus for the initial seven sessions. In the remaining nine sessions, a rational-emotive therapy approach was used to modify maladaptive cognitions. In addition, stress inoculation procedures were used to promote generalization of relaxation skills. The aim of these sessions was to develop stress management skills as active coping strategies for dealing with symptoms at home and on the job. The intervention targeted at maladaptive cognitions included identification of activating events (symptoms and environmental stimuli), associated cognitive appraisals as related to health, and the emotional and environmental consequences of such beliefs. Self-monitoring tasks were provided to identify the associations among symptoms, thought processes, and emotions.

At termination R. L. reported symptom-free days but continued to report minimal symptoms (such as heartburn) on an average of two days per week. The patient reported that he had returned to work and was maintaining a regular exercise program (jogging fifteen to twenty minutes a day, five times per week) and resuming social activities. Anxiolytic medication (Xanax) was reduced from .5 mg three times a day to .5 mg once a day; however, the use of Deseryl and Lopressor continued at initially prescribed levels. In sum, the patient complied with treatment procedures and reported changes in mood and behavior. Follow-up at six-week intervals was scheduled.

Conclusions

Evaluation and treatment of arrhythmias from a bio-behavioral perspective involve a set of procedures designed to identify and modify environmental, psychological, behavioral, and psychophysiological factors assumed to contribute to the etiology, exacerbation, and maintenance of the disorder. Such an approach requires a careful consideration of the medical aspects of the case, including pathophysiology and ongoing pharmacological management. The biobehavioral techniques employed should be carefully integrated with medical management; that is, the referring physician should periodically evaluate the effects of such techniques on the arrhythmia of concern.

Biobehavioral intervention is usually targeted at anxiety/stress, depression/somatization, and health risk behavior. Treatment protocols often involve time-limited programs (fifteen to thirty one-hour sessions) for the anxiety and depression components, with follow-up visits representing an essential aspect of patient management, particularly for the initial eighteen months. Effective health risk modification usually requires longer-term efforts and continuous involvement in a structured program (such as an aerobic dance class).

Much of the material presented in the "Treatment Protocol" section of this chapter represents our own clinical approach to arrhythmias. The literature evaluating the effects of various biobehavioral approaches on specific forms of arrhythmia remains quite limited. Therefore, it is difficult to generate a specific list of treatment suggestions and prognostic indicators that are based on an empirical literature. As indicated elsewhere (Feuerstein and Ward, 1980), there continues to be a paucity of large-scale, well-controlled, long-term outcome studies evaluating the differential effects of biobehavioral techniques with and without medication. In addition, there are no empirical studies to guide clinical decisions on whether or when the consulting cardiologist should reduce medication in patients receiving concurrent biobehavioral treatment. This should clearly be the decision of the cardiologist, and a close working relationship between the behavioral medicine specialist and the cardiologist is essential.

From a diagnostic perspective, the use of ambulatory psychophysiological monitoring continues to hold much promise in identifying event-related arrhythmias, perhaps permitting in the future a more sophisticated choice of treatment options. Yet we are not aware of any published work on the use of this approach in the biobehavioral assessment of the arrhythmia patient. Clearly, such research would be most promising.

In sum, the biobehavioral approach to arrhythmias has proceeded beyond the heart rate biofeedback technique frequently reported in the past decade to an approach that appears more integrative. Such an approach, as represented in the present chapter, incorporates a variety of techniques with diverse goals related to the patient's pattern of presenting problems. While such an integrative approach has been useful clinically, and each of the techniques has been supported in clinical investigations with various clinical samples, the approach has not been exposed to the rigors of a clinical trial in patients with arrhythmias. Until that time, despite its apparent clinical value, such an approach can serve only as a preliminary protocol.

References

Ackerman, S. H., and Sachar, E. J. "The Lactate Theory of Anxiety: A Review and Re-Evaluation." *Psychosomatic Medicine*, 1974, *36*, 69–81.

American Psychiatric Association. *Diagnostic and Statistical Manual of Mental Disorders.* (3rd ed.) Washington, D.C.: American Psychiatric Association, 1980.

Apfel, R., and Sifneos, P. E. "Alexithymia: Concept and Measurement." *Psychotherapy and Psychosomatics,* 1979, *32,* 180-190.

Barchas, J. D., and others (Eds.). *Psychopharmacology: From Theory to Practice.* New York: Oxford University Press, 1977.

Barsky, A. J., and Klerman, G. L. "Overview: Hypochondriasis, Bodily Complaints, and Somatic Styles." *American Journal of Psychiatry,* 1983, *140,* 273-283.

Beck, A. T. *Cognitive Therapy and the Emotional Disorders.* New York: International Universities Press, 1976.

Beck, A. T., and others. *Cognitive Therapy of Depression.* New York: Guilford Press, 1979.

Bellet, S. *Clinical Disorders of the Heart Beat.* (3rd ed.) Philadelphia: Lea & Febiger, 1971.

Benson, H., Alexander, S., and Feldman, C. L. "Decreased Premature Ventricular Contractions Through Use of the Relaxation Response in Patients with Stable Ischaemic Heart Disease." *Lancet,* 1975, *2,* 380-382.

Bigger, J. T. "Mechanisms of Arrhythmias." In E. Braunwald (Ed.), *Heart Disease: A Textbook of Cardiovascular Medicine.* Philadelphia: Saunders, 1980.

Blanchard, E. B., and Abel, G. G. "An Experimental Case Study of the Biofeedback Treatment of a Rape-Induced Psychophysiological Cardiovascular Disorder." *Behavior Therapy,* 1976, *7,* 113-119.

Bleecker, E. R., and Engel, B. T. "Learned Control of Ventricular Rate in Patients with Atrial Fibrillation." *Psychosomatic Medicine,* 1973a, *35,* 161-175.

Bleecker, E. R., and Engel, B. T. "Learned Control of Cardiac Rate and Cardiac Conduction in the Wolff-Parkinson-White Syndrome." *New England Journal of Medicine,* 1973b, *288,* 560-562.

Bove, A. A. "The Cardiovascular Response to Stress." *Psychosomatics,* 1977, *18* (4), 13-16.

Braunwald, E. (Ed.). *Heart Disease: A Textbook of Cardiovascular Medicine.* Philadelphia: Saunders, 1980.

Brownell, K. D. "The Addictive Disorders." In C. M. Franks and others (Eds.), *Annual Review of Behavior Therapy: Theory and Practice.* New York: Guilford Press, 1982.

Carroll, B. J. "The Dexamethasone Suppression Test for Melancholia." *British Journal of Psychiatry*, 1982, *140*, 292-304.

Chapman, R. A., and Miller, D. J. "The Effects of Caffeine on the Contraction of the Frog Heart." *Journal of Physiology*, 1974, *242*, 589-613.

Ciminero, A. R., Calhoun, K. S., and Adams, H. E. (Eds.). *Handbook of Behavioral Assessment*. New York: Wiley-Interscience, 1977.

Clarke, J. M., and others. "The Rhythm of the Normal Human Heart." *Lancet*, 1976, *2*, 508-512.

Collison, D. R. "Cardiological Applications of the Control of the Autonomic Nervous System by Hypnosis." *American Journal of Clinical Hypnosis*, 1970, *12*, 150-156.

Dahlstrom, W. G., Welsh, G. S., and Dahlstrom, L. E. *An MMPI Handbook*. Vol. 2: *Clinical Interpretation*. Minneapolis: University of Minnesota Press, 1975.

Davidson, P. O., and Davidson, S. M. (Eds.). *Behavioral Medicine: Changing Health Lifestyles*. New York: Brunner/Mazel, 1980.

Dobmeyer, D. J., and others. "The Arrhythmogenic Effects of Caffeine in Human Beings." *New England Journal of Medicine*, 1983, *308*, 814-816.

Ellis, A., and Abrahams, E. *Brief Psychotherapy in Medical and Health Practice*. New York: Springer, 1978.

Engel, B. T., and Bleecker, E. R. "Application of Operant Conditioning Techniques to the Control of Cardiac Arrhythmias." In P. A. Obrist and others (Eds.), *Cardiovascular Psychophysiology*. Hawthorne, N.Y.: Aldine, 1974.

Ferrer, M. I. "Sick Sinus Syndrome." *Circulation*, 1973, *47*, 635-641.

Feuerstein, M., and Ward, M. M. "Psychological Treatment of Cardiac Arrhythmias." In J. M. Ferguson and C. B. Taylor (Eds.), *The Comprehensive Handbook of Behavioral Medicine*. Vol. 1. Jamaica, N.Y.: SP Medical & Scientific Books, 1980.

Fielding, J. E. "Effectiveness of Employee Health Improvement Programs." *Journal of Occupational Medicine*, 1982, *24*, 907-916.

Fowler, N. O. *Cardiac Arrhythmias: Diagnosis and Treatment.* (3rd ed.) New York: Harper & Row, 1980.

General Health Incorporated. *Health Self-Appraisal Report.* Washington, D.C.: General Health Incorporated, 1977.

Gilbert, D. G., and Haggen, R. L. "The Effects of Nicotine and Extroversion on Self Report, Skin Conductance, Electromyographic and Heart Rate Responses to Emotional Stimuli." *Addictive Behaviors,* 1980, *5,* 247-257.

Gruen, W. "Effects of Brief Psychotherapy During the Hospitalization Period on the Recovery Process in Heart Attacks." *Journal of Consulting and Clinical Psychology,* 1975, *43,* 223-232.

Hackett, T. P., and Rosenbaum, J. F. "Emotion, Psychiatric Disease, and the Heart." In E. Braunwald (Ed.), *Heart Disease: A Textbook of Cardiovascular Medicine.* Philadelphia: Saunders, 1980.

Hinkle, L. E., Carver, S. T., and Stevens, M. "The Frequency of Asymptomatic Disturbances of Cardiac Rhythm and Conduction in Middle-Aged Men." *American Journal of Cardiology,* 1969, *24,* 629-650.

Jarvik, M. E. "Biological Influences on Cigarette Smoking." In *Smoking and Health: A Report of the Surgeon General.* DHEW Publication No. 79-50066. Washington, D.C.: U.S. Government Printing Office, 1979.

Kallman, W. M., and Feuerstein, M. "Psychophysiological Procedures." In A. R. Ciminero, K. S. Calhoun, and H. E. Adams (Eds.), *Handbook of Behavioral Assessment.* New York: Wiley-Interscience, 1977.

Kallman, W., and Feuerstein, M. "Psychophysiological Procedures in Behavior Therapy, Behavioral Medicine, and Neuropsychology." In A. R. Ciminero, K. S. Calhoun, and H. E. Adams (Eds.), *Handbook of Behavioral Assessment.* (2nd ed.) New York: Wiley-Interscience, in press.

Katz, L. N., and Pick, A. *Clinical Electrocardiography.* Part 1: *The Arrhythmias.* Philadelphia: Lea & Febiger, 1956.

Katz, L. N., Winton, S. S., and Megibow, R. S. "Psychosomatic Aspects of Cardiac Arrhythmias: A Physiological Dynamic Approach." *Annals of Internal Medicine,* 1947, *27,* 261-274.

Kostis, J. B., and others. "Ambulatory Electrocardiography: What Is Normal?" (Abstract.) *American Journal of Cardiology,* 1979, *43,* 420.

Lesser, I. M. "A Review of the Alexithymia Concept." *Psychosomatic Medicine,* 1981, *43,* 531–543.

Levine, B. J., and others. "Lack of Correlation Between Symptoms and Significant Arrhythmias on Long-Term Electrocardiographic Analysis." *Clinical Research,* 1978, *26,* 247A.

Lewinsohn, P. M., Sullivan, J. M., and Grosscup, S. J. "Behavioral Therapy: Clinical Applications." In A. J. Rush (Ed.), *Short-Term Psychotherapies for Depression.* New York: Guilford Press, 1982.

Lown, B., and DeSilva, P. A. "Roles of Psychologic Stress and Autonomic Nervous System Changes in Provocation of Ventricular Premature Complexes." *American Journal of Cardiology,* 1978, *41,* 979–985.

Lown, B., Verrier, R., and Corbalan, R. "Psychologic Stress and Threshold for Repetitive Ventricular Response." *Science,* 1973, *182,* 834–836.

Lown, B., Verrier, R., and Rabinowitz, S. H. "Neural and Psychologic Mechanisms and the Problem of Sudden Cardiac Death." *American Journal of Cardiology,* 1977, *39,* 890–902.

Lown, B., and others. "Basis for Recurring Ventricular Fibrillation in the Absence of Coronary Heart Disease and Its Management." *New England Journal of Medicine,* 1976, *294,* 623–629.

Lynch, J. J., and others. "Human Contact and Cardiac Arrhythmia in a Coronary Care Unit." *Psychosomatic Medicine,* 1977a, *39,* 188–192.

Lynch, J. J., and others. "Psychological Aspects of Cardiac Arrhythmia." *American Heart Journal,* 1977b, *93,* 645–657.

MacKay, C. "The Measurement of Mood and Psychophysiological Activity Using Self-Report Techniques." In I. Martin and P. H. Venables (Eds.), *Techniques in Psychophysiology.* New York: Wiley, 1980.

Martin, J. E., and Dubbert, P. M. "Exercise Applications and Promotion in Behavioral Medicine: Current Status and Future Directions." *Journal of Consulting and Clinical Psychology,* 1982, *50,* 1004–1017.

Meichenbaum, D. *Cognitive-Behavior Modification: An Integrative Approach.* New York: Plenum, 1977.

Meichenbaum, D., and Cameron, R. "Stress Inoculation Training: Toward a General Paradigm for Training Coping Skills." In D. Meichenbaum and M. E. Jaemko (Eds.), *Stress Reduction and Prevention.* New York: Plenum, 1983.

Milsum, J. H. "Lifestyle Changes for the Whole Person: Stimulation Through Health Hazard Appraisal." In P. O. Davidson and S. M. Davidson (Eds.), *Behavioral Medicine: Changing Health Lifestyles.* New York: Brunner/Mazel, 1980.

Moos, R. H. (Ed.). *Coping with Physical Illness.* New York: Plenum, 1977.

Moos, R. H. *Work Environment Scale Manual.* Palo Alto, Calif.: Consulting Psychologists Press, 1981.

Moos, R. H., and Moos, B. S. *Family Environment Scale Manual.* Palo Alto, Calif.: Consulting Psychologists Press, 1981.

Nietzel, M. T., and Bernstein, D. A. "Assessment of Anxiety and Fear." In M. Hersen and A. S. Bellack (Eds.), *Behavioral Assessment: A Practical Handbook.* (2nd ed.) Elmsford, N.Y.: Pergamon Press, 1981.

Ostrander, L. D., and others. "Electrocardiographic Findings Among the Adult Population of a Total Natural Community, Tecumseh, Michigan." *Circulation,* 1965, *31,* 888-898.

Phibbs, B. *The Cardiac Arrhythmias.* (3rd ed.) St. Louis: Mosby, 1978.

Pickering, T. G., and Gorham, G. "Learned Heart Rate Control by a Patient with a Ventricular Parasystolic Rhythm." *Lancet,* 1975, *1,* 252-253.

Pickering, T. G., and Miller, N. E. "Learned Voluntary Control of Heart Rate and Rhythm in Two Subjects with Premature Ventricular Contractions." *British Heart Journal,* 1977, *39,* 152-159.

Pilowsky, I., and Spence, N. D. "Illness Behavior Syndromes Associated with Intractable Pain." *Pain,* 1976, *2,* 61-71.

Pitts, F. N., and McClure, J. N. "Lactate Metabolism in Anxiety Neurosis." *New England Journal of Medicine,* 1967, *277,* 1329-1336.

Prineas, R. J., and others. "Coffee, Tea and VPB." *Journal of Chronic Diseases,* 1980, *33,* 67-72.

Rahe, R. H., and Christ, A. E. "An Unusual Cardiac (Ventricular) Arrhythmia in a Child: Psychiatric and Psychophysiologic Aspects." *Psychosomatic Medicine,* 1966, *28,* 181-188.

Rahe, R., and Romo, M. "Recent Life Changes and the Onset of Myocardial Infarction and Sudden Death in Helsinki." In E. Gunderson and R. Rahe (Eds.), *Life Stress and Illness.* Springfield, Ill.: Thomas, 1974.

Ray, W. J., and Raczynski, J. M. "Psychophysiological Assessment." In M. Hersen and A. S. Bellack (Eds.), *Behavioral Assessment: A Practical Handbook.* (2nd ed) Elmsford, N.Y.: Pergamon Press, 1981.

Regestein, Q. R. "Relationships Between Psychological Factors and Cardiac Rhythm and Electrical Disturbances." *Comprehensive Psychiatry,* 1975, *16,* 137-148.

Rehm, L. P. "Assessment of Depression." In M. Hersen and A. S. Bellack (Eds.), *Behavioral Assessment: A Practical Handbook.* (2nd ed.) Elmsford, N.Y.: Pergamon Press, 1981.

Rodnick, J. E. "Health Behavior Changes Associated with Health Hazard Appraisal Counseling in an Occupational Setting." *Preventive Medicine,* 1982, *11,* 583-594.

Rosenbaum, M. "A Schedule for Assessing Self-Control Behaviors: Preliminary Findings." *Behavior Therapy,* 1980, *11,* 109-121.

Rush, A. J. (Ed.). *Short-Term Psychotherapies for Depression.* New York: Guilford Press, 1982.

Scott, R. W., and others. "A Shaping Procedure for Heart Rate Control in Chronic Tachycardia." *Perceptual and Motor Skills,* 1973, *37,* 327-338.

Silver, B. V., and Blanchard, E. B. "Biofeedback and Relaxation Training in the Treatment of Psychophysiological Disorders: Or Are the Machines Really Necessary?" *Journal of Behavioral Medicine,* 1978, *1,* 217-239.

Stoyva, J., and Budzynski, T. "Cultivated Low Arousal: An Antistress Response?" In L. V. DiCara (Ed.), *Limbic and Autonomic Nervous System Research.* New York: Plenum, 1974.

Trautwein, W. "Membrane Currents in Cardiac Muscle Fibers." *Physiological Reviews,* 1973, *53,* 793-835.

Wagner, E. H., and others. "An Assessment of Health Hazard/ Health Risk Appraisal." *American Journal of Public Health,* 1982, *72*, 347–352.

Weiss, T., and Engel, B. T. "Operant Conditioning of Heart Rate in Patients with Premature Ventricular Contractions." *Psychosomatic Medicine,* 1971, *33*, 301–321.

Young, J. E., and Beck, A. T. "Cognitive Therapy: Clinical Applications." In A. J. Rush (Ed.), *Short-Term Psychotherapies for Depression.* New York: Guilford Press, 1982.

Zifferblatt, S. M., and Wilbur, C. S. "Maintaining a Healthy Heart: Guidelines for a Feasible Goal." *Preventive Medicine,* 1977, *6*, 514–525.

3

Cardiac Surgery:
Enhancing
Postoperative Outcomes

Larry S. Goldman, M.D.
Chase Patterson Kimball, M.D.

Few medical interventions have more captured the fascination and hope of both those with heart disease and the public at large than has cardiac surgery. It is the stuff of high drama, as perhaps the most psychologically symbolic organ is exposed and manipulated. Each year in the United States, more than 175,000 persons—ranging from newborns with life-threatening congenital anomalies to octogenarians whose heart walls have softened and bulged out (forming ventricular aneurysm) following a heart attack—undergo cardiac surgery. In 1982 a mechanical heart was implanted for the first time in the chest of a man whose own heart muscle was failing to pump adequately to sustain his life. Unfortunately, he died, but his determined struggles were followed daily for months by an avid public.

113

Yet each surgical procedure is not only an amazing feat of technology; for the person undergoing it, it is a profound life experience. Each patient brings a unique set of biological and psychological strengths and vulnerabilities to the operation, a set of variables that profoundly shape the experience, the complications, the long-term success, and even the risk of death. This chapter seeks to convey to health and mental health professionals what these variables and experiences are and to devise a rational plan of interventions to optimize the experiences and the benefits, not only medically but psychologically as well.

The Disorders

Like any major organ, the heart may exhibit a host of malfunctions seen in clinical practice. The interested reader should consult several standard references for more than the necessarily superficial discussion here (Anderson, 1971; Lev, 1958; Netter, 1969). In general, surgery on the heart is considered in cases where discrete anatomical lesions have led to compromised cardiovascular physiological functioning. An attempt is made to restore as much anatomical integrity as possible (for instance, to sew up a bullet wound or to replace a badly damaged valve with an artificial one).

Coronary Artery Disease. The coronary arteries are relatively small blood vessels that arise from the root of the aorta (that is, where it joins the heart) and provide the blood supply to the heart muscle itself. Clearly, any compromise in the functioning of these vessels may compromise the heart's supply of nutrients and oxygen and thus its ability to function. Narrowing of the vessels is caused by fatty deposits over the years (atherosclerosis) or by blood clots. Patients with these lesions may have heart attacks (actual death of muscle tissue) and/or periodic transient compromises in the blood flow, leading to chest pain (angina pectoris). Sometimes vessel narrowing leads to decreased contractility of the heart, with shortness of breath the prominent symptom. Further description of coronary artery disease can be found in Chapter Four.

A variety of medical treatments are available for angina,

but some patients are refractory to these. In addition, certain critical types of obstructions in the vessels are known to carry an excessive risk of mortality if left untreated. Obstruction of the left main coronary artery, a lesion often referred to as a "widow maker," carries a 63 percent risk of death within six years (Corday, 1975). For these and for other situations that are more controversial, coronary artery bypass grafts (CABGs) are performed. This surgery consists of replacement of diseased arteries with grafts taken from the saphenous veins of the legs (Favalaro and others, 1970). Most patients undergoing such surgery are middle-aged or older and frequently have histories of angina, heart attacks, and sometimes strokes. Many have been ill for several years with progressively worsening symptoms, and they arrange surgery at their own convenience; others may have a first attack of angina and be emergently rushed to surgery if critical lesions and imminent cardiac compromise are found.

    Cardiac Valve Disease. The heart contains four valves, which ensure the orderly flow of blood from two large blood vessels (the vena cava and the pulmonary vein) to two large vessels (the pulmonary artery and the aorta). Adequate functioning of the valves requires adequate patency (to allow blood flow in the desired direction) and competency (to prevent backflow of blood in the wrong direction). A number of diseases can damage these valves. The most common is rheumatic fever (a hypersensitivity reaction that occasionally follows certain streptococcal infections), which causes thickening, scarring, and rigidity of one (usually the mitral) or more valves. Another frequent cause of damage is endocarditis, in which infections in the bloodstream cause the growth of vegetations on valve leaflets.

    Patients experience a variety of symptoms depending on the site(s) and type(s) of damage. Shortness of breath (dyspnea), particularly with exertion, cyanosis (blue skin), and syncopal (fainting) episodes are particularly common. Occasionally pieces of vegetation from a damaged valve may become dislodged and propelled into the circulation. These can cause strokes or blockage of blood vessels leading to other organs. Since rheumatic heart disease often has its onset in childhood but may display only a slow evolution of symptoms, patients might be well into young adulthood or even middle age before they go to surgery. Thus, some of these patients have a particularly long history of experiencing themselves as sick, a history that spans numerous developmental milestones.

Congenital Anomalies. The various cardiac anomalies can differ in severity. Common ones are atrial septal defects (ASDs) and ventricular septal defects (VSDs), both of which result in backflows of oxygenated blood from the left side of the heart to the right. Other lesions include obstructions, interpositions, or transpositions of the main blood vessels leading to or from the heart. Major disorders are treated early in life and are not discussed here. Minor anomalies may not yield symptoms (usually exertional dyspnea) or signs (murmurs, cyanosis) until later in life.

Other Conditions. Cardiac surgery is used less commonly for a number of other situations, including repair of trauma to the heart, biopsies, excision of tumors, repair of aneurysms, ablation of electrical conduction fibers, removal of a diseased pericardium (the lining around the heart), and so on.

The Surgery

The details of surgery vary from center to center and with the procedure being done. The patient is anesthetized and a variety of monitoring devices attached: a thermometer, an intra-arterial catheter to measure blood pressure, a bladder catheter to collect and measure urine output, a catheter in the pulmonary artery to measure pressure, and electrocardiographic heart leads to record heart rhythm. A tube is passed into the trachea to assist breathing.

The chest is then opened, usually via an incision along the breastbone or occasionally in the side of the chest. If a coronary artery surgery is being performed, several veins are removed from the patient's leg. Since the heart's pumping activity would be impeded by the subsequent manipulations, the large vessels are attached to a heart-lung machine ("the pump"), which will assume this activity. At this point the patient's heart is no longer sustaining his life. Then the major procedure is done. This may be the replacement of the diseased coronary arteries with the venous grafts, the incision of the heart itself (actual "open-heart" surgery) to replace valves or patch a graft over a septal defect, the oversewing of an aneurysm, and so on. The heart is then detached from the pump (usually with bated breath), and it resumes its regular beating activity. The suture lines are checked, and if all is well, the chest is closed with a chest tube in place to drain fluid and maintain the lungs in an expanded state. The operation lasts several hours.

The Recovery

The patient moves from the surgical suite to the recovery room. Upon awakening he finds all the aforementioned instruments in place. Thus, he cannot speak. There is pain in the incision site, particularly with inspiration, and there may be pain or discomfort at the insertion sites of several tubes. If he remains stable, he is transferred to a Cardiac Surgery Intensive Care Unit (CSICU), where he will remain for four or more days in the company of fellow sufferers under intense medical and nursing surveillance. It is here that there is a constant risk of abnormal heart rhythms, blood clots, strokes, heart attacks, pneumonia, wound infections, and many other problems. Periodically a patient stops breathing or his heart stops beating, and he must be resuscitated.

Eventually the patient is transferred to a less restrictive, less closely supervised setting. Most catheters have been removed, but the heart rhythm is usually monitored for a few more days. Pain abates and ambulation is encouraged. The patient may spend up to a few more weeks in the hospital and then be given instructions for home care.

Some Preoperative Considerations

A number of elements pertinent to preoperative care will be clarified in the next section, as postoperative outcomes are traced back to preoperative risk factors; but a few points are made here for emphasis and because they do not follow quite so directly.

Many cardiologists and cardiac surgeons deliberately or automatically make some psychological assessment of surgical candidates and often find no cause for concern. The patient's response to investigative procedures may often presage what occurs during and after surgery, and so is worth observing carefully. Several specific manifestations should give concern and indicate the need for psychiatric screening:

1. *Depression.* Several authors (Kennedy and Bakst, 1966; Kimball, 1969) have drawn attention to the increased risk of medical complications and death in these patients, who may allow surgery as a passive suicide attempt. Vigorous treatment may be needed, and delay of surgery is occasionally advisable.

2. *Cognitive dysfunction.* The presence of cognitive deficits, whether in a clear or a clouded state of consciousness, also presages difficulty, not only medically but also in increased risk of postoperative psychosis (see next section). If no treatment can be provided, careful observation before and after surgery is warranted.

3. *Marked ambivalence.* While some ambivalence is quite normal when one is contemplating cardiac surgery, it may occasionally indicate a familial conflict where the patient feels pressured into surgery. Covert messages of negation (multiple postponements, last-minute development of unexplained symptoms) may be the clues.

4. *Questionable cardiac findings.* Many people have symptoms suggestive of cardiac disease but no physical pathology. A patient eager for surgery with equivocal examination results may suffer from a primarily psychiatric illness (Kennedy and Bakst, 1966). Somatic delusions ("My heart is filled with bugs") as part of a psychotic illness (schizophrenia or depression generally), conversion disorder (Engel, 1969), and surgery-seeking behavior to resolve unconscious guilt (Menninger, 1934; Engel, 1959) are common findings. These disorders should of course be treated psychiatrically rather than surgically.

In general, patients with these conditions, with the possible exception of those who have a severe cognitive dysfunction, are technically capable of giving informed consent, since the disorders do not interfere with their ability to comprehend the risks of surgery. Nonetheless, informed consent generally requires some explanation of the prognosis of the untreated condition as well as of alternative forms of therapy (Miller, 1980); and a patient's understanding of these factors may be materially affected by his psychiatric condition. Thus, the markedly depressed surgical candidate may pessimistically see prognosis and medical management as quite hopeless when they may not be, while viewing the risk of dying at surgery as a preferable alternative. One could argue that legally this constitutes informed consent, but the ethical position is far more ambiguous.

The Psychological Experience of Cardiac Surgery

In a society fascinated by technology, the technical aspects of cardiac surgery have claimed much of the attention, but only a few moments of consideration can allow a thoughtful observer to realize the staggering psychological implications of the process as well. A person with a longstanding illness, which has restricted his life and which may well progress and even threaten his life, becomes faced with the opportunity to arrest and remedy much of the illness. But of course the price is a high one: The patient must allow a group of relative strangers to break open his chest, stop his heart's functioning while various maneuvers are performed on and around it, and restart the heart; endure a prolonged convalescence marked by pain, restriction of activities, enforced passivity, sensory over- and understimulation, and the ongoing risk of sudden disaster; and, finally, begin a rehabilitation designed to undo perhaps decades of limitations on his life. It is clear that navigating these waters would be a tremendous task for even the most "adjusted" person.

Although the many aspects of this experience could easily fill this chapter, five major themes are virtually ubiquitous and are described at length in the literature.

Risk of Death. This primordial and yet realistic fear

permeates the patient's thinking from the time surgery is first contemplated, and it may persist for long after surgery. Although the fear of dying may be regarded as a fundamental existential condition (Yalom, 1980), what is seen clinically is the mobilization of additional fears (such as castration anxiety) and the defenses erected against the anxiety so created. Blacher and Cleveland (1979, p. 2464) discuss a forty-five-year-old woman whose intense fear of death prevented her from agreeing to much-needed surgery. During a psychiatric interview, the patient realized a previously repressed fantasy: that when her heart would be stopped during surgery, she would have the opportunity to go to heaven to rejoin her long-dead and much-missed father. Understanding this conflict about joining him or returning to life allowed her to proceed with surgery.

An example of extreme defensive operations is provided by Kennedy and Bakst's (1966, p. 840) description of "a most infantile forty-two-year-old spinster" whose sister had recently died during cardiac surgery. During preoperative evaluations the patient simulated fever by rubbing her thermometer and later developed hysterical total-body anesthesia. Of some note here is that the patient died of a fatal arrhythmia on the night of surgery after her family insisted on the surgery over initial psychiatric objections.

More commonly, patients handle death anxiety by varying amounts of denial, displacement ("No, I'm just worried about her driving to the hospital to see me in all that traffic"), or counterphobic behavior (such as unusual risk-taking activities). Interestingly, there is an almost universal belief that the risk of dying from surgery is 50–50, regardless of the figure presented by the surgeon (Blacher and Cleveland, 1979).

Sense of Awe. Beyond its life-sustaining physiological function, the heart performs a central symbolic role in the emotional life as well. One hears this in many figures of speech: heart of the matter, a broken heart, losing heart, losing one's heart to another person, and so on. Thus, as Blacher (1972, p. 305) eloquently describes, there is a nearly universal sense of awe in the notion that one's heart will be handled, stopped, and incised. He reports that almost all patients initially react to this notion with denial, but that the awe may surface shortly after surgery, when the danger is passed. He cites Edington's (1969, p. 163) observation that brighter, more alert patients may be at increased risk of developing postoperative delirium and speculates that this may be in part due to such patients' increased openness to the awe reaction.

Postoperative Environment. The patient awakening from anesthesia, no matter how well prepared before surgery, finds himself in a distinctly surrealistic situation. Even if he has been extubated and can speak, he finds numerous other devices going into and emerging from a variety of body orifices. The cardiac monitor beeps with each heartbeat, the oxygen hisses into his mask, and in the background respirators click with unceasing regularity. The room is usually lit with fluorescent lighting, and there may be few clues (such as windows or clocks) to reveal the time of day (or night). Movement is limited by pain and tubing. Doctors and nurses patrol, speaking in whispered tones. Periodically some catastrophe occurs, and medical staff rush to a bedside while new noises (such as thumping) are heard. Attempts to sleep are punctuated by interruptions for checks of vital functions. This environment is the patient's life for several days until he is ready for transfer from the intensive care unit.

The effect of all this on the patient is disquieting at best and frequently disorienting. Kornfeld, Zimberg, and Malm (1965, p. 291) have drawn attention to the similarities between this environment and those reported in sleep and sensory deprivation studies (West and others, 1962; Solomon and others, 1961; Fiskind and others, 1963), as well as the parallels between the psychoses of postoperative patients and of subjects exposed to such deprivations. The disruptions of sleep, the absence of orienting cues, the monotonous background noises punctuated by unexpected sounds, and the mechanical rather than human emphasis provide alternating sensory overload and understimulation, which promote hypnoid and psychotic-like states.

Another set of difficulties concerns the patient's relations with his caregivers. Although the patient realizes that requests (or demands) from nurses to move, breathe deeply, and

allow suctioning or percussion are well intended, they also increase his physical discomfort. Since the patient's very life depends on these ministrations, he must find ways of dissipating
the anger engendered by these contacts. The projection of such
anger is a fairly common paranoid solution adopted by some patients (Blacher and Cleveland, 1979).

As time progresses, physical comfort becomes less problematic, and the need for care from nurses diminishes. It is then
that the patient's characterological difficulties with such issues
as enforced passivity, dependency, and loss of control may become manifest; and open conflicts may arise between patient
and staff, with attempts at splitting (dividing staff into "all
good" and "all bad" people and playing one group against the
other), acting out, and power struggles (Cassem and Hackett,
1971). These disruptions may begin after a few days in the ICU
if the patient's course has been a medically smooth one, but
they most commonly become manifest about the time of transfer to the general floor. This transition from intense personal
and mechanical surveillance to a setting of diminished observations is considered to be "flying on one's own" or "sink or
swim" by patients, and so anxiety and defensive operations increase in this vulnerable period (Klein and others, 1968).

Survivor Guilt. Blacher (1978) and Blacher and Cleveland
(1978) noticed a number of patients who developed a depression beginning a number of days after surgery, usually at the
point where it seemed that the patient could expect a smooth
course. They discovered that these "paradoxical depressions"
were caused by the patient's guilt over surviving an illness that
had taken the life of one or more family members who had not
undergone surgery. Presenting the conflict to the patient and
discussing the excessive guilt led to rapid resolution of the depression.

Change in Status. Eventually the patient's medical recovery ends, and he must now adapt to a life with new valves, coronary arteries, and so on. For many patients the reduction in
symptoms and improvement in function was the highly desired
goal for which they had made the sacrifice of surgery. But it is
not an easy transition to go from being sick to being well after

years or perhaps even decades of disability. Changes in work roles, recreation, sex, and personal relationships all become necessary. Most patients, who regarded their cardiac disease as an enemy, can mourn the loss of their old lives readily and move on. But others have grown addicted to the sick role. For these the prospect of working, playing, and living their lives fully means relinquishing the dependency, passivity, and diminished responsibilities to which they have grown accustomed (Kasl and Cobb, 1964, 1966). If the patient's social system has made the sick role an acceptable or even a pleasant one, then both the system and the patient must change after surgery. Those patients who cannot change retain their old symptoms even when objective criteria say they should not, or they develop new symptoms. In these cases correction of lesions is only a Pyrrhic victory, and the disappointment and anger felt by the patient (who usually is not consciously aware of his "addiction") spreads rapidly to his family and doctors as well.

Postoperative Delirium

The vast majority of the publications on psychiatric aspects of cardiac surgery in the past thirty years have focused on the predominant clinical problem in the field—namely, the extraordinarily high incidence of severe postoperative mental disturbances. About one patient in 1,500 undergoing general surgery develops a psychosis postoperatively (Knox, 1961), yet as many as 70 percent of those patients undergoing open-heart surgery may experience a delirium following surgery (Kornfeld, Zimberg, and Malm, 1965). This section will review the literature on this topic, emphasizing risk factors and areas of potential intervention, and it will conclude with some of the strategies for prevention and management.

In 1954 Fox, Rizzo, and Gifford reported that 19 percent of a group of patients undergoing mitral commisurotomy developed a variety of severe psychological disturbances following surgery. All subsequent investigators have verified that cardiac surgery yields an unusually high incidence of such disturbances, which have been described by a wide range of labels: psychoses, delirious states, confusional states, disruptions, severe behavioral disorders, agitation, paranoia, and disorientation, among others. Although these terms may be accurate descriptions of particular patients' states, the lack of agreement on terminology, including the use of different definitions for the same term (such as delirium) in different reports, has in some instances made it difficult to compare findings and explore the etiology of the entire phenomenon. Since most case descriptions involve some change in the level of the patient's consciousness, perceptual disturbances, disorientation, fluctuation over time, and brief course, the term "delirium" will be used here, as it is by most authors, but it should be borne in mind that not all cases are technically delirium (American Psychiatric Association, 1980; Engel and Romano, 1959).

Several reports soon confirmed the findings of Fox, Rizzo, and Gifford. Bliss, Rumel, and Branch (1955) reported a 16 percent incidence of postoperative disorders after closed-heart surgery; Kaplan (1956), 17 percent; Meyer, Blacher, and Brown (1961), 13 percent. This last group described "catastrophic reactions," characterized by a rigid, motionlessness posture and an appearance of terror or apathy. Other authors found lower incidences: Bolton and Bailey (1956), 3.1 percent; Knox (1963), 4.4 percent; and Dencker and Sendahl (1961), 4.9 percent.

There seemed to be a trend toward lower incidences in later studies, which was subsequently noted with open-heart surgery as well. This was probably a function of (1) improved technical quality of the procedures and postoperative care over time, (2) recognition and reduction of risk factors shown by research to be related to delirium, and (3) possibly the confounding presence of psychological researchers themselves, which may have affected the progress of some patients.

On the other hand, early studies generally used chart review to identify disordered cases, a definite methodological flaw. Kornfeld, Zimberg, and Malm (1965) found an incidence by chart review of 38 percent postoperative disorders, a figure that climbed to 70 percent in a subgroup of patients actually interviewed. Similarly, Blacher (1972) challenged ICU nurses to identify patients who "showed no evidence of emotional difficulty"; eight of the patients selected revealed that they had had postoperative psychotic experiences. Thus, later studies (which generally utilized patient interviews rather than chart review or nursing reports) might have been expected to find higher incidences of postoperative delirium than earlier studies.

In 1964 both Blachly and Starr and Egerton and Kay published reports documenting even higher incidences of postoperative delirium following open-heart surgery (for valve or congenital anomaly repair) than for closed-heart procedures, 57 percent and 41 percent respectively. Subsequent reports over the next thirteen years revealed incidences of 13 to 51 percent (Dubin, Field, and Gastfriend, 1979), most reports suggesting that one quarter to one third of patients are affected. Even taking into account the factors of patient selection, case identification, and differing definitions, it is clear that the incidence is dramatically high.

According to the classical descriptions of this "postcardiotomy delirium" (Blachly and Starr, 1964), a lucid period for several days after surgery is followed by a relatively rapid onset of perceptual distortions, progressing to delusions and secondary behavioral disturbances (for example, attempts to flee from imaginary persecutors). The syndrome lasts several days, with some cases persisting for up to a few weeks. A typical case is the following:

Mr. M., a forty-eight-year-old married father of two without previous psychiatric history, was electively admitted for repair of a mitral valve damaged by rheumatic heart disease. He was quiet but cooperative for forty-eight hours after surgery but then became preoccupied with the hissing of the oxygen tubes. He noticed the nurses whispering rather than talking while making rounds, and he gradually came to realize that they were pumping "female hormones" into his "oxygen." He repeatedly removed his mask and quarreled with the nurses about replacing it. He demanded to see the doctor on the fourth postoperative night, but he interpreted the sleepy on-call resident's behavior as furtive and became convinced that the resident was part of the plot. Mr. M. disconnected his monitor and threatened to leave. He was sedated and the next morning transferred from the ICU to the monitored floor. Within twelve hours his psychosis and his agitation had cleared.

A number of variations of this "classical" picture have been described. Kimball (1969) called attention to the presence of delirious states beginning immediately after surgery without a lucid interval, as well as to a "euphoric reaction," which seemed to occur more commonly in patients with hysterical traits. This reaction might be akin to a manic defense. As mentioned, Meyer, Blacher, and Brown (1961) described a "catastrophic" response similar to that noted by Goldstein (1951) in his work with brain-damaged patients or to that of Engel's (1962) conservation-withdrawal state. It remains unestablished whether these descriptions refer to different conditions or whether they are variable presentations of a single underlying syndrome.

Similar disturbances were found following coronary artery bypass surgery. In 1975 Rabiner, Willner, and Fishman reported a 16 percent incidence of delirium postoperatively. Subsequent reports by Sveinnson (1975), Kornfeld and associates (1978), and Katz (1978) yielded figures of 12, 28, and 29 percent respectively.

Risk Factors. Most studies that examined the relation between age and risk of delirium found a statistically significant correlation or at least a positive trend (Blachly and Starr, 1964; Rabiner, Willner, and Fishman, 1975; Weiss, 1966; Tufo, Ostfeld, and Shekelle, 1970; Layne and Yudofsky, 1971; Heller and others, 1970; Surman and others, 1974), although a few did not (Bolton and Bailey, 1956; Kornfeld, Zimberg, and Malm, 1965; Rubinstein and Thomas, 1969; Lee and others, 1971). Three studies suggest an increased risk for males (Blachly and Starr, 1964; Layne and Yudofsky, 1971; Henrichs and Waters, 1972), one for females (Rubinstein and Thomas, 1969), and seven found no relation (Bolton and Bailey, 1956; Kornfeld, Zimberg, and Malm, 1965; Heller and others, 1970; Lee and others, 1969; Freyhan and others, 1971; Surman and others, 1974; Rabiner, Willner, and Fishman, 1975). So it seems most likely that increasing age increases the risk while sex does not.

The occurrence of delirium in children is considered to be quite rare. Children have been less studied than adults, but there have been enough reports to support this conclusion, which has been explained on both physiological (decreased risk of neurological damage from surgery) and psychological (lack of full awareness of concept of death) grounds.

A number of reports have examined the relationship between postoperative delirium and severity of cardiac disease, either by New York or American Heart Association criteria. The results have been equivocal. No relation was found in five studies (Bolton and Bailey, 1956; Egerton and Kay, 1964; Javid and others, 1969; Tufo, Ostfeld, and Shekelle, 1970; Henrichs, MacKenzie, and Almond, 1971); and a positive correlation was found in four (Blachly and Starr, 1964; Heller and others, 1970; Kornfeld, Zimberg, and Malm, 1965; Freyhan and others, 1971). Longer duration of heart disease (Kornfeld, Zimberg, and Malm, 1965; Henrichs, MacKenzie, and Almond, 1971) and rheumatic valvular as opposed to congenital or coronary artery disease (Blachly and Starr, 1964; Egerton and Kay, 1964; Heller and others, 1970; Burgess, Kirklin, and Steinhilber, 1967; Willner and others, 1976) both seem to increase the risk.

Considerable evidence exists to implicate preoperative central nervous system (CNS) dysfunction as a potent risk factor. Priest and associates (1957), using psychometric testing, found exacerbations of preoperative perceptual organic deficits following surgery in patients with rheumatic heart disease. Tufo, Ostfeld, and Shekelle (1970) found that a history of neurological deficits did not correlate with postoperative cerebral damage but that the presence of neurological deficits was a strong correlate of behavioral disturbances. Heller and colleagues (1970) found preoperative organicity (established by EEG, interview, and psychometric testing) to be related to early postoperative delirium but not to the "classical" delirium occurring after a lucid period. Kimball (1972)—using the Wechsler Adult Intelligence Scale, block design tests, and an interview—found a high incidence of preoperative organicity, and such organicity correlated with ICU disorientation (as well as postoperative medical complications and risk of death). Other authors further support the role of preoperative CNS dysfunction as a potent risk factor for postoperative disturbances (Willner and others, 1976; Branthwaite, 1972; Kornfeld and others, 1974).

A variety of operative factors has shown a relationship to the likelihood of postoperative delirium. These include the length of time of the bypass pump run (longer pump time predicts greater risk of delirium), use of profound hypothermia (Silverstone, Tannahill, and Ireland, 1970), hypotension (less than 50-60 mm Hg), and type of procedure (generally, multiple valve > single valve > congenital anomaly > bypass graft > closed-heart valve repair) (Heller and others, 1978). Data on other operative factors—such as total duration of the operation, type of anesthesia, perfusion flow rate, or disk versus bubble oxygenator—are too equivocal or inadequate to permit any conclusions to be drawn.

Postoperative conditions have, somewhat surprisingly, been less studied than pre- and intraoperative factors. Heller and his associates (1970) developed a physical sickness rating scale from 1 to 4, with mean scores of 3.5 for patients developing early delirium, 2.5 for "classical" delirium, and 1.4 for no-delirium patients. In general, conditions that might predispose to delirium in any setting—conditions such as decreased cardiac output (Blachly, 1967), acute renal failure (Blachly and Kloster, 1966), arrhythmias, hypoxemia, and use of barbiturates—seem to make delirium more likely after cardiac surgery. Hazan (1966a, 1966b) has speculated that one or more psychotoxic amines might be released during surgery and yet not cause a reaction until a few days later, when cardiac output is returning to normal and the hypothesized amines have become well circulated. Unfortunately, such amines have never been documented. Lee and colleagues (1971) did note a rise in catecholamines postoperatively but without any correlation with delirium, and Abram (1971) states that these toxins have yet to be found.

Other investigators have called attention to the link between postoperative delirium and neurological factors. Autopsy studies of patients who died after cardiac surgery have revealed a high incidence of ischemic changes consistent with hypotension or microemboli (Tufo, Ostfeld, and Shekelle, 1970; Javid and others, 1969). Many patients with postoperative behavioral disturbances have exhibited focal neurological signs (Gilman, 1965) or EEG changes (Kornfeld, 1967; McKegney, 1966). The number of patients studied both neurologically and psychiatrically has been small, so that these reports are merely suggestive and not conclusive.

Abram (1971) and Kornfeld, Zimberg, and Malm (1965) were the first to call attention to the atmosphere of the recovery room and the surgical intensive care unit as a factor that might contribute to postcardiotomy delirium. They noted the "sensory-monotony experience" (Solomon and others, 1961) brought on by immobility and the continuous background noises of hissing oxygen tubing and beeping cardiac monitors. The effect of this "white noise" is to lull the patient into a hypnoid or semiwakeful state, which renders him less able to integrate other sensory input. Thus, alterations in ward activity or behaviors of ward personnel are dimly perceived, with the attendant risk of minor or even gross misperceptions. The use of sedatives, narcotic analgesics, and hypnosis probably aggravates this state as well. Furthermore, the patient's attempts to sleep are interrupted by checks of vital signs, buzzers, the noise of nursing shift changes, and other events. That many patients with delirium clear shortly after transfer from the CSICU also implies an important causal role of these factors.

A number of studies have investigated the role of premorbid (presurgical) personality and life-stressor factors on the development of postoperative delirium. Early reports were primarily anecdotal and often retrospective, inferring conflicts from the content of psychotic material. Subsequent studies used interviews and/or psychological testing preoperatively to match with postsurgical outcome.

Dencker and Sandahl (1962) and Egerton and Kay (1964) found a higher incidence of serious mental illness in patients who developed delirium than in those who did not. Egerton and Kay also found a higher rate of disturbed marriages and of personal problems unrelated to surgery in the delirious group. On the other hand, Blachly and Starr (1964) found a higher incidence of both preoperative psychiatric disturbance (33 percent) and disrupted home life (27 percent) in patients who did *not* develop delirium, as opposed to those who did (19 percent and 8 percent are the comparable figures). Kornfeld, Zimberg, and Malm (1965) were also unable to find differences in marital status between the two groups. Finally, Rubinstein and Thomas (1969) found that 54 percent of their patients assigned a preoperative psychiatric diagnosis developed a delirium, while 17 percent of those without such a diagnosis did.

Similarly conflicting results were found by investigators using standard psychological testing. Henrichs and Waters (1972) and Henrichs, MacKenzie, and Almond (1969) administered the Minnesota Multiphasic Personality Inventory (MMPI) to a group of preoperative patients. This test measures a variety of personality traits and components (Dahlstrom, Welsh, and Dahlstrom, 1975). Henrichs and his colleagues found no difference in MMPI profiles between males who did and those who did not develop postoperative delirium. Weiss (1966) found differences for both sexes. In a relatively small sample, Gilberstadt and Sako (1967) found no difference in preoperative MMPI profiles between subsequently delirious and nondelirious patients. Shealy and Walker (1978) obtained the same result with a larger sample. Kornfeld and colleagues (1974) found that patients "characterized by dominance, aggressivity, and self-assuredness" as measured on the Cattell and Eber (1957) 16 Personality Factor Questionnaire were more likely to develop delirium. They hypothesized that from a psychological viewpoint such patients might have special difficulty tolerating the enforced postoperative passivity. Although these personality traits also correlated with length of intraoperative pump time, another factor thought to increase the risk of developing delirium, Kornfeld and his associates cite the report of Cohen and Lazarus (1973) to support their belief that personality was the primary factor.

Kennedy and Bakst (1966) intensively studied a group of

136 patients, whom they divided into six groups based on pre-operative interviews:

Group I: Strongly motivated to become healthy; flexible use of denial to minimize fear.
Group II: Superficially eager for health but actually disease-dependent to avoid normal role.
Group III: Conflicted about recovery, panicky about prospects of surgery.
Group IV: Also ambivalent but more afraid of recovery than of surgery; often pressured into surgery.
Group V: Unconscious wish to die, "sanctioned suicide."
Group VI: No real cardiac disease, primarily psychiatric illness causing symptoms.

The highest incidence of postoperative delirium was found in Group III (51 percent), while none was found in Group VI. Groups I, II, IV, and V had rates of 28, 33, 41, and 33 percent, respectively. A number of patients in Groups II and IV had *pre*-operative psychiatric disturbances, and 55 percent of patients in Group II and 47 percent in Group IV died postoperatively. Thus, high levels of preoperative anxiety seemed to predispose to delirium, while large amounts of secondary gain from illness predicted preoperative psychoses and higher mortality after surgery.

Kimball (1969) devised a similar grouping into four categories, but the overall low incidence of postoperative disturbances in his study precluded conclusions based on these groupings. Nonetheless, he was able to document excess mortality in patients in groups described as "anxious" and "depressed," as opposed to "adjusted" or "symbiotic." In a later study designed to look more closely at postoperative behavior, Kimball (1970) did find a correlation between confusion and both low overt anxiety and dependency. Layne and Yudofsky (1971) confirmed that low preoperative anxiety seems to predict a higher risk of postoperative psychosis.

It is clear from the above discussion that a host of factors can be shown to correlate with the development of postcardiac surgery psychosis and delirium but that no one factor or set of factors has primacy. In 1971 Abram urged an end to conflict between "organicists" and proponents of a strictly psychological model. Since such disparate factors as bypass pump time, preoperative neurological deficits, interpersonal dominance, and sensory monotony in the recovery room are (among others) predictors of such a state, a more integrated biopsychosocial model, such as that of Lipowski (1967) or Engel (1977), seems called for. The postoperative states under discussion are best conceptualized as final common pathways for the sum of cognitive, emotional, physical, and environmental factors. That no single factor can be singled out may disturb unitarists, but the complexity of the phenomenon means that a variety of interventions may be clinically useful.

Intervention. A small number of studies have been published on the effects of preoperative interventions on the risk of postoperative delirium. Meyer, Blacher, and Brown (1961) posited from their uncontrolled data that intervention reduces this risk. In 1967 Burgess, Kirklin, and Steinhilber studied three groups of patients: two control groups and an intervention group that received a preoperative psychiatric interview (and also postoperative follow-up). The incidences of postoperative disturbances were 16.7 percent and 35.4 percent in the two control groups and 27.8 percent in the intervention group. This study, which does not demonstrate that intervention is beneficial, was flawed because the researchers failed to establish comparable groups and used retrospective chart data to establish the presence of delirium. This second problem also marred the study of Lazarus and Hagens (1968), who found a 33 percent incidence of postoperative psychosis at a control hospital and 14 percent at a hospital (used by the same surgeons) where patients had a preoperative interview.

Layne and Yudofsky (1971) compared two groups of patients undergoing cardiac surgery: eighteen patients who received standard preoperative care and a neurological evaluation and forty patients who also underwent "an extensive interview" the evening before surgery. They reported a significantly lower rate (10 percent versus 22 percent, $p < .05$) of postoperative psychoses in their intervention group. Kornfeld and associates (1974) confirmed this finding, demonstrating a halved incidence (7 percent versus 14 percent) of delirium in patients who received a preoperative interview lasting one and a half to three hours. Once again, however, in Kornfeld's study the presence of delirium was established by chart review, and the authors mention that personal interviews in the experimental group postoperatively established a 25 percent incidence of delirium.

A methodologically more sound study was reported by Surman and associates (1974), who compared two carefully matched groups of patients undergoing mitral valve surgery. Patients in the experimental group received a preoperative interview and were taught autohypnosis. Both groups were followed postoperatively to assess mental status. To the authors' surprise, there was no statistically significant difference between their experimental and control groups in the incidence of delirium, which they defined very broadly. There also was no difference between groups in postoperative pain, anxiety, or use of analgesic, anxiolytic, or sedative drug use. The authors raise the question of whether hypnosis might increase the risk of delirium.

Finally, Aiken and Henrichs (1971) compared a group of patients taught systematic relaxation (Wolpe and Lazarus, 1966) with a control group. Although they found a decrease in delirium in the intervention group, this group also differed significantly from the control group in a number of intraoperative variables thought to be implicated in the risk of postoperative delirium.

Thus, although, as discussed later, there may be some benefits from preoperative psychological interventions, reducing the risk of delirium has not been conclusively shown to be one of them.

Surprisingly, the management of postoperative psychoses has been little studied, and most authors' recommendations have been heuristic or anecdotal rather than carefully evaluated. In general, the approach to the patient is the same as that for any delirium: early diagnosis, search for contributing medical

factors, environmental manipulation, and judicious pharmaco-
therapy (Hackett and Cassem, 1978).

Early diagnosis is important because an incipient state
can be aborted and complications (such as disconnected lines or
patient falls) avoided. Clues to the onset of delirium include
hypervigilance (Kimball, 1969), forgetfulness, lability of mood,
and illusions or other perceptual disturbances. An increased
amount of psychological care with opportunities for patient
ventilation, reassurance, and correction of misperceptions may
arrest the progression (Freyberger, 1978). Particular attention
should be paid to pain and anxiety, since inadequate or over-
zealous prescribing of narcotics or anxiolytics may aggravate the
situation.

The form of delirium may give important clues to some
of the psychological (conflictual) factors contributing to it.
Thus, as a first approximation, "frozen" patients exhibiting the
"catastrophic" type of disorder might well be approached as if
they were terrified of death, and this topic could be a focus of
an interview. Similarly, patients exhibiting paranoid trends may
be harboring angry and counterdependent feelings, both subjects for psychological exploration. Finally, patients having
"euphoric" reactions may be warding off depression or fears of
catastrophe. Of course, such psychotherapeutic approaches will
be more useful early or in milder cases; the grossly agitated patient in little contact is in no condition to reflect on his anxieties.

Although we have been emphasizing the multifactorial
etiology of postcardiac surgery delirium, a search for the usual
causes of, or contributing medical factors to delirium also must
be made. Changes in mental status are often the first indication
of neurological insults, pulmonary emboli, hypotension, sepsis,
renal failure, electrolyte imbalances, hypoxemia, and a host of
other derangements that may later become more apparent. Correction or amelioration of such disorders may rapidly (as in
hypotension) or more slowly (as in hyponatremia) improve or
cure the disorder.

Kornfeld, Zimberg, and Malm (1965) were perhaps the
first to make discrete recommendations about environmental
manipulations to reduce the risk of or improve the disordered

mental state. Their suggestions include (1) allowing as much sleep as possible and attempting to maintain the usual sleep-wake cycle; (2) keeping monitoring devices outside the patient's hearing, both to reduce the monotony and to avoid anxiety about changes in the devices; (3) minimizing the noise of oxygen and air conditioning; (4) protecting patients from witnessing emergency procedures or deaths of other patients (although, of course, staff should almost always explain or reveal to patients who do ask); and (5) increasing sensory cues and stimuli (at appropriate times) by the presence of clocks, calendars, radios, television, and frequent brief visits by nursing personnel. Similar recommendations have been made by other authors as well (McKegney, 1966; Nadelson, 1976). Attention should be paid in particular to patients with sensory deficits (Weisman and Hackett, 1958) or those who are not English speaking (Danilowicz and Gabriel, 1971).

The mainstay of pharmacological intervention is clearly the class of drugs known as antipsychotics or neuroleptics (Blachly and Starr, 1966). Currently the most useful of these drugs in an ICU setting is the butyrophenone haloperidol, a drug with far fewer anticholinergic and alpha-adrenergic-blocking effects than other neuroleptics. Thus, it minimizes the risk of tachycardia, urinary retention, ileus, and hypotension commonly seen with some other antipsychotics (Davis and Casper, 1977). In particular, Sos and Cassem (1978) have demonstrated minimal or no changes in heart rate, systolic blood pressure, pulmonary artery pressure, pulmonary wedge pressure, cardiac rhythm, ECG, or respiratory rate in postcardiac surgical patients given up to 25 mg (a relatively large dose) as an intravenous bolus and up to 185 mg intravenously over twenty-four hours. They recommend a strategy of progressively increasing doses at thirty-minute intervals in a loading regimen until sedation is achieved, with subsequent administration of 50 percent of the total loading dose twelve hours later. Maintenance would be continued orally or intravenously (using bedtime dosages) for up to a few days after the clearing of the delirium. Although they report no extrapyramidal side effects, haloperidol does have potent dopamine-blocking effects, and one must watch for the occurrence of dystonia, akathisia (which may appear as increased patient restlessness), and akinesia (which may appear as "psychomotor retardation" or "depression") (Henn, 1982; Davis and Casper, 1977).

Summary. Few today would fail to agree that the incidence of severe psychiatric disturbances following cardiac surgery is quite high compared to other surgical procedures and that the causes are multiply determined. In general, older and physically sicker patients with preoperative cognitive or neurological deficits are at increased risk, probably independently of their psychological makeup. Open-heart operations with increased pump times and more hypotension increase the risk. A variety of postoperative medical complications and environmental variables may provide fertile ground for the germination of delirium. Attention to improvement of these factors, early recognition, increased psychological supportive care, and appropriate drug usage are the mainstays of management. Preoperative psychological interventions have not been consistently shown to have a prophylactic value, but they do of course establish the basis of a therapeutic relationship, which may be utilized following surgery.

Other Postoperative Problems

As the previous section has demonstrated, the immediate postoperative period is a time of great risk of serious psychiatric disturbance, occasionally subtle but not infrequently dramatic as well. The medical issues of morbidity and mortality and the psychophysiological one of delirium dominate the picture. But other problems are also important during the ICU phase—namely, pain and anxiety and, during the post-ICU phase, depression and disruption. While a large body of data exists on the management of postcardiac surgery delirium, much less has been written about these four problems as they pertain to this patient population. Thus, clinicians must rely on conclusions reached in other settings, such as medical ICUs and coronary care units. These problems will be reviewed briefly here.

Pain. In a now classic study, Egbert and co-workers

(1964), using a double-blind strategy, showed that preoperative instructions provided by the anesthesiologist regarding what to expect, how to relax, and how to breathe and move reduced patients' need for postoperative analgesics by almost half. Healy (1968) also demonstrated a reduced need for analgesia in a group of general surgical patients given special instructions on breathing, moving, and expectations, as compared to a control group receiving "routine" care. Sime's (1976) study of fifty-seven women admitted for abdominal surgery demonstrated that the level of preoperative fear correlated with the amount of postoperative analgesia. One can infer that steps taken to reduce anxiety might well have an effect on this variable. The Surman (1974) study with cardiac surgery patients did not demonstrate this type of effect, but intervention there took the form of teaching autohypnosis rather than preparing the patient and providing education. A recent meta-analysis by Mumford, Schlesinger, and Glass (1982), reviewing thirty-four controlled studies of surgical patients receiving preoperative information and/or support, revealed a mean improvement effect size of .44 for pain reduction and .1, for lowered analgesic use, a powerful indicator of the effect of intervention. (Effect size reflects the average difference between control and intervention patients on a scale standardized by dividing the actual rating by the standard deviation of the control group.) Thus, in addition to the judicious use of drugs (Marks and Sachar, 1973) and hypnosis postoperatively, a preoperative discussion with the patient involving coming events, teaching of relaxation exercises, and provision of instructions on movement and breathing can also be expected to reduce pain.

    Anxiety. As discussed earlier, anxiety frequently parallels the patient's clinical condition after surgery. Excessive symptoms of anxiety should always raise the question of an organic (usually cardiopulmonary) etiology, such as pulmonary embolus or arrhythmias (Dietch, 1981), or the mobilization of unconscious conflicts, usually around passivity, dependency, or autonomy. Mumford, Schlesinger, and Glass (1982) found discernible benefits of preoperative intervention on both pre-operative and postoperative measures of anxiety (patient self-ratings). Anticipating bloody drainage from a chest tube is a far cry better than suddenly noticing it unprepared.

Finally, it is worth repeating that, while the use of anxiolytics may be most efficacious for the short-term management of anxiety, their potential contribution to postoperative delirium and the small risk of paradoxical excitement must be borne in mind.

Depression. It seems odd that depression might follow a procedure designed to improve the quality of life, but it does occur. Patients with protracted postoperative courses marked by multiple complications may evidence demoralization, characterized by a conservation-withdrawal response (Engel, 1980) or a hopeless-helpless stance (Engel and Schmale, 1967). Reassurance based on facts (as opposed to wishful thinking) and the instillation of hope are the mainstays of intervening in this problem. On the other hand, "paradoxical depression," a term coined by Blacher (1978) and described earlier in this chapter, is a product of survivor guilt. This conflict-based depression needs to be elucidated and the unreasonable superego (conscience) response confronted.

A depressive reaction may be seen in some patients contemplating the changes in their lives that might be brought about by surgery. This may be regarded as a normal grieving process (Lindemann, 1944) for an old self-concept (that of a sick person) and lifestyle. If mild, it is probably the beginning of a necessary adaptive process and should be explained to the patient as such, so that he can tolerate the affect and understand the positive implication of the process.

The use of antidepressant medication is rarely warranted in postoperative depressions. In addition to the augmented risk of serious side effects in this patient population, two to three weeks may need to elapse before a response is observed. Although some of the newer antidepressants are touted as having fewer side effects and a quicker onset of action, these claims have yet to be rigorously established. For the rare patient with a profound depression (particularly with a high risk of suicide), stimulants or electroconvulsive treatment (ECT) may be quicker acting, safer, and more efficacious (American Psychiatric Association, 1978).

Disruption. Cassem and Hackett (1971), in their report on psychiatric consultation in a coronary care unit (CCU), noted a multimodal pattern of referrals for post-MI management problems. The group of patients seen early in the hospitalization exhibited considerable anxiety or denial, manifested as threats to sign out or sexual provocation of the nurses. The group seen (on the average) a few days later exhibited hostile-dependent conflicts, usually of a passive-aggressive nature. The authors felt that the second group represented patients with longstanding interpersonal difficulties who had been "paralyzed" with fear for a few days but then resumed their difficult styles. Since cardiac surgery patients generally volunteer for surgery, denial in these forms is seldom seen, but the mobilization of character problems after physical danger is over is not uncommon.

These patients are often best handled by a psychiatric consultant, who can combine support for the patient's anxieties with tactful confrontation about the patient's behavior. The consultant may also serve as a lightning rod for the patient's and the staff's anger, and he may provide much-needed support for the staff caring for such "hateful" or otherwise difficult patients (Groves, 1975, 1978). Staff may deal initially with such patients by attempting to set limits on their behavior; but the main difficulty is that the patients—because of the hostility that they engender and experience—may perceive such limit setting (or even the consultation) as motivated by vengeful rather than therapeutic intent.

Rehabilitation

Assessing the long-term effects of cardiac surgery is a task fraught with ambiguities and methodological obstacles. Direct interviews of patients (and spouses) probably yield the most reliable data, but many patients are understandably not eager to cooperate. Questionnaires yield better response rates, but it is impossible to avoid the biases inherent in incomplete returns and the subjectivity of the responders. But what constitutes a good outcome? To the surgeon and the cardiologist, reduction in symptoms and a move to normalization of physiological meas-

ures may indicate success. Yet one can question the degree of
success if intractable angina or exertional dyspnea is relieved by
surgery but the patient continues to restrict his life as before.
On the other hand, for some patients whose newly created coronary arteries demonstrate obstruction soon after surgery, symptoms remain absent and functioning improves. In spite of all this
uncertainty, a fair amount of research has been done, and some
tentative conclusions can be drawn.

Knox (1963) interviewed a group of eighty-three patients
three years after they had undergone mitral valve surgery.
About three fifths had good results; but the remainder displayed depression, anxiety, hysterical symptoms, poor medical
outcome, or cognitive deficits. The patients with these symptoms had been more negatively affected by their cardiac disease
before the operation and were more dependent and sexually
maladjusted than those in the good outcome group.

Kimball (1969) interviewed thirty-eight survivors of
open-heart surgery at two-month intervals for three to fifteen
months after surgery. Before surgery he had classified these patients into four groups: adjusted, symbiotic, anxious, and depressed. He reported a 75 percent improvement rate in the adjusted group, 7 percent in the symbiotic, no consistent pattern
of outcome in the anxious, and no improvement or a worsening
in all the depressed survivors. It should be added that in this
study 75 percent of the depressed group and 25 percent of the
anxious group had died perioperatively.

Lucia and McGuire (1970) found generally good vocational, social, and psychological functioning in a group of one
hundred patients responding by questionnaire three years after
valve surgery. Yet in a larger questionnaire survey (263 patients), Blachly and Blachly (1968) found that 41 percent of
the patients felt unable to work, and 39 percent felt "worse off"
when asked how the operation had affected their "nerves."
Nonetheless, 97 percent of the patients felt that they had benefited from surgery, and 58 percent reported an improved "out-
look on life." Almost 800 of 1,100 members of the Mended
Hearts Society responded to questionnaires by Frank, Heller,
and Kornfeld (1972) an average of about six years after cardiac

surgery. Some 96 percent of the patients were glad they had had surgery, and three quarters felt psychologically better in the year following surgery. Half to three quarters reported improvements in job performance, mood, family relations, nervousness, and sexual relations at one year postoperatively. The remainder reported no change in these variables or some worsening (3 to 13 percent).

Burgess, Kirklin, and Steinhilber (1967) found that about one quarter of their patients surveyed a year after surgery had poor psychological outcomes, including somatization, depression, anxiety, and behavioral disturbances. Of some interest was their finding that patients whom they had interviewed during the hospital course fared considerably better than those who were not interviewed.

Several investigators have tried to determine whether postoperative delirium is associated with a poorer long-term prognosis. Heller and associates (1974) found in a one-year follow-up of patients who had undergone open-heart valvular surgery a sizable proportion of patients with psychological hindrances to recovery, but such hindrances correlated strongly with preoperative maladjustment rather than postcardiotomy delirium, cardiac status, or postoperative life stresses. Rabiner and Willner (1976) reached similar conclusions about the relationship between immediate postoperative psychopathology and long-term psychological functioning in a group of patients eighteen months after coronary artery bypass surgery. Only the study by Henrichs, MacKenzie, and Almond (1971) suggested otherwise, but their conclusions were based on inferences from MMPI results at six months, and the relationship was noted only in males.

More recent reports have examined outcomes following coronary artery surgery. In a group of thirty patients interviewed before surgery and one to two years later, Gundle and associates (1980) found generally good physiological outcome but high unemployment (83 percent) and sexual dysfunction (57 percent). Both of these outcomes were correlated with preoperative duration of cardiac symptoms and with preoperative level of functioning in each area. The authors acknowledged that their high unemployment rate could in part be explained by the lower socioeconomic status of their patients compared to others (blue-collar workers generally need more physical capabilities than white-collar), but they noted work inhibition even in patients who were physically capable of working.

In a larger study, Anderson and associates (1980) found that return to work after bypass surgery was a function of patient age and that 90 percent of the patients younger than fifty-five at the time of surgery had returned to work four years later. Twenty-two percent of patients not employed before surgery were employed at the four-year follow-up. This finding confirmed the findings of Symmes, Lenkei, and Berman (1978) but contradicted those of Barnes and his co-workers (1977). In a recent study (Jenkins and others, 1983), 318 bypass patients were interviewed and asked to fill out questionnaires six months after surgery. The investigators found highly positive outcomes on both physical and psychological measures, including diminished anxiety, depression, fatigue, and insomnia. Three quarters of the employed patients returned to work, and half to two thirds reported no changes in their marital relationship. Although these findings are encouraging, it is important to realize that these patients were healthier as a group than the group of all patients in the United States undergoing open-heart surgery (for instance, they had no other illnesses, and they had not had previous cardiac surgery). Moreover, a minority of patients did not fare so well.

Finally, Brown and Rawlinson (1979) compared social and psychological functioning in a group of patients randomly assigned to medical or surgical therapy for chronic stable angina. Nine or more months after the patients had enrolled in the study, no differences between the patients treated medically and those undergoing surgery were found in work status, social activity, family functioning, life satisfaction, or anxiety. Medically treated patients did, however, report more depression.

What can one conclude from this literature? In general, it seems that most patients undergoing cardiac surgery derive psychological, social, and vocational benefits from it. Nonetheless, a sizable minority of patients report or exhibit work inhibition, interpersonal difficulties, sexual dysfunction, hysterical symptoms, anxiety, or depression. These patients seem to be those who exhibited preoperative maladjustment in their lives. There is some suggestion that longer disability before surgery may increase the risk of rehabilitation problems, since the more chronically sick patients may have been more habituated to a "sick role" (Parsons and Fox, 1952). Patients exhibiting marked dependency, depression, or denied anxiety may be at particular risk of poor outcome. These findings seem to apply to both open- and closed-heart valve repair, coronary artery surgery, and probably congenital anomaly repair as well, in spite of the fact that duration of illness and age at onset certainly differ between patients undergoing each type of surgery.

Only one study examined an intervention (Burgess, Kirklin, and Steinhilber, 1967), finding that psychiatric interviews throughout the hospitalization improved the long-term outcome. In the absence of validating studies, this finding must be regarded as tentative. Nonetheless, preoperative identification of patients with psychological risk factors for poor results ought to be undertaken and attempts made to prevent such outcomes. A psychotherapeutic strategy designed to highlight fears and conflicts about change in roles seems most promising. Such a strategy would include realistic reassurances about what to expect and how to cope with impending changes, as well as some exploration of unconscious anxieties when they seem paramount.

Change in longstanding characterological problems cannot, of course, be effected during a several-week hospitalization, but a combined educative and behavioral approach, using interpretations at periods of blockage (resistance), may have profound effects, as it has had in the treatment of sexual dysfunctions (Kaplan, 1974). An example:

Mrs. R., a forty-two-year-old mother of two, was admitted for repair of mitral valve damage caused by rheumatic heart disease when she was twelve. She had been working as a sociology professor until two years earlier, when dyspnea limited her ability to lecture. Preoperatively she revealed a clinging, almost symbiotic relationship with her husband much as she had with her mother. She reported that, after the death of her brother when she was eleven years old, she and her mother had drawn together.

The patient seemed ambivalent about the surgery in spite of her marked physical symptoms. She smiled as she complained about her inability to work. Initial focus was on allowing her to acknowledge the extent of her anxiety about surgery. As she did so, she revealed that her brother had been killed in an automobile accident on his way to a movie, which she had refused to see with him. She realized that she had regarded her heart disease as appropriate punishment for her "negligence" toward her brother.

Postoperatively she did poorly, developing many unexplained symptoms. Gradually she began to realize that she was reluctant to become well because then she would not be cared for. Her symptoms abated as she understood this, and she began to talk about her husband's resentment of her work and his preference that she remain home. Several interviews with the patient and her husband clarified that her beliefs about his feelings were her projections.

Six months after surgery, the patient had resumed work and was granted tenure. She reported occasional vague chest pains when her husband left town on business, but she said, "I know what those mean."

There is considerable evidence to suggest that clinically depressed patients fare extremely poorly at cardiac surgery, with a grossly excessive rate of mortality and of serious medical complications. Those who survive the postoperative course seem unlikely to benefit much from the surgery. Such patients should, whenever clinically possible, have surgery postponed while treatment for the depression is instituted. Just as a good surgeon would not operate on a patient with poorly controlled hypertension or diabetes, he should also hesitate to operate on a seriously depressed patient.

Transplants, Artificial Hearts, and Beyond

There have been three waves of cardiac surgery: closed-chest valve repairs, open-heart procedures, and coronary artery bypass surgery. Each has been heralded as the latest application of modern medical technology, and each has benefited a different set of patients. Yet, curiously enough, the psychological problems have remained much the same: anticipatory fear, postoperative delirium, pain, and rehabilitation, as well as others discussed in this chapter. Only the numbers and perhaps the nuances seem to change. Early observers of cardiac transplants, a procedure now perhaps about to undergo a renaissance because of improved immunosuppressive drugs, described in their small group of patients the same problems faced by other cardiac surgery patients (Kraft, 1971; Lunde, 1969). Additional psychological difficulties face any transplant recipient, particularly one who undergoes cardiac transplantation (see Castelnuovo-Tedesco, 1971). Recently, for example, newspaper accounts described the postoperative delirium of Barney Clark, recipient of the world's first artificial heart.

This seemingly paradoxical situation of changing technology and more static psychology can be resolved by appreciation of the parallels in the patient's experience of each of these types of surgery. A person with "heart disease," whether fixed or progressive, thinks of himself as "a sick person," especially as symptoms worsen over time. A major surgical assault is undertaken to correct the lesion(s), subjecting the circulatory, pulmonary, and central nervous systems to a variety of insults. The patient's postoperative state is characterized by pain, immobility, dependency, sensory monotony, and ongoing risk of disaster. Finally, the medical pitfalls are overcome, and he now faces a life that will be dramatically different from his previous way of living.

Thus, new technology can certainly be expected to bring more of the same biopsychosocial difficulties. While it will be important to anticipate the psychological impact of such experiences as having an artificial heart permanently pumping one's blood, or receiving a heart from a suicide victim, there are today still some unanswered questions about the reactions in patients undergoing current surgeries. These are mainly in the area of effective intervention, such as whether neuroleptics do alter the course of a delirium, whether preoperative evaluation and preparation are helpful or necessary, or whether in-hospital interventions affect the long-term results. Many studies using sound methodologies (control groups, blindness, randomization, and the like) have already answered many questions in this field about phenomenology and etiology, but therapeutics have been less extensively addressed.

Psychosocial research has always been the "poor relation" in medical settings, not only because of its "softness" (the absence of meaningfully quantitative variables) but because much of the early work was vague and impressionistic. It is clear now that psychological interventions may affect such "hard" variables as length of hospital stay, rate of employment, and even mortality. More rigorous, controlled designs are increasingly finding their way into such research, and many of the questions raised in this chapter may eventually be answered by these designs. Future cardiac patients can "take heart" from the research both done and yet to come.

References

Abram, H. S. "Psychotic Reactions After Cardiac Surgery: A Critical Review." *Seminars in Psychiatry,* 1971, *3,* 70–78.

Aiken, L. H., and Henrichs, T. F. "Systematic Relaxation as a Nursing Intervention Technique with Open Heart Surgery Patients." *Nursing Research,* 1971, *20,* 212–217.

American Psychiatric Association. *Electroconvulsive Therapy.* Task Force Report 14. Washington, D.C.: American Psychiatric Association, 1978.

American Psychiatric Association. *Diagnostic and Statistical Manual of Mental Disorders.* (3rd ed.) Washington, D.C.: American Psychiatric Association, 1980.

Anderson, A. J., and others. "Retention or Resumption of Employment After Aortocoronary Bypass Operations." *Journal of the American Medical Association,* 1980, *243,* 543–545.

Anderson, W. A. D. (Ed.). *Pathology*. (6th ed.) St. Louis: Mosby, 1971.

Barnes, G. K., and others. "Changes in Working Status of Patients Following Coronary Bypass Surgery." *Journal of the American Medical Association*, 1977, *238*, 1259–1262.

Blacher, R. S. "The Hidden Psychosis of Open-Heart Surgery: With a Note on the Sense of Awe." *Journal of the American Medical Association*, 1972, *222*, 305–308.

Blacher, R. S. "Paradoxical Depression After Heart Surgery: A Form of Survivor Syndrome." *Psychoanalytic Quarterly*, 1978, *47* (2), 267–283.

Blacher, R. S., and Cleveland, R. J. "Paradoxical Depression After Heart Surgery." In H. Speidel and G. Rodewald (Eds.), *Psychic and Neurological Dysfunctions After Open-Heart Surgery*. New York: Thieme-Stratton, 1978.

Blacher, R. S., and Cleveland, R. J. "Heart Surgery." *Journal of the American Medical Association*, 1979, *242* (22), 2463–2465.

Blachly, P. H. "Open-Heart Surgery: Physiological Variables of Mental Functioning." *International Psychiatry Clinics*, 1967, *42*, 133–155.

Blachly, P. H., and Blachly, B. J. "Vocational and Emotional Status of 263 Patients After Heart Surgery." *Circulation*, 1968, *38*, 524–533.

Blachly, P. H., and Kloster, F. E. "Relation of Cardiac Output to Post-Cardiotomy Delirium." *Journal of Thoracic and Cardiovascular Surgery*, 1966, *52*, 422–427.

Blachly, P. H., and Starr, A. "Post-Cardiotomy Delirium." *American Journal of Psychiatry*, 1964, *121*, 371–375.

Blachly, P. H., and Starr, A. "Treatment of Delirium with Phenothiazine Drugs Following Open-Heart Surgery." *Diseases of the Nervous System*, 1966, *27*, 107–110.

Bliss, E. L., Rumel, W. R., and Branch, C. H. H. "Psychiatric Complications of Mitral Surgery." *Archives of Neurology and Psychiatry*, 1955, *74*, 249–252.

Bolton, E. B., and Bailey, C. P. "Psychosomatic Aspects of Cardiovascular Surgery: Surgical Aspects." In A. J. Cantor and

A. N. Foxe (Eds.), *Psychosomatic Aspects of Surgery.* New York: Grune & Stratton, 1956.

Branthwaite, M. A. "Neurological Damage Related to Open-Heart Surgery: A Clinical Survey." *Thorax,* 1972, *27,* 748–753.

Brown, J. S., and Rawlinson, M. E. "Psychosocial Status of Patients Randomly Assigned to Medical or Surgical Therapy for Chronic Stable Angina." *American Journal of Cardiology,* 1979, *44,* 546–554.

Burgess, G. N., Kirklin, J. W., and Steinhilber, R. M. "Some Psychiatric Aspects of Intracardiac Surgery." *Mayo Clinic Proceedings,* 1967, *42,* 1–12.

Cassem, N. H., and Hackett, T. P. "Psychiatric Consultation in a Coronary Care Unit." *Annals of Internal Medicine,* 1971, *75,* 9–14.

Castelnuovo-Tedesco, P. "Organ Transplant, Body Image, Psychosis." In P. Castelnuovo-Tedesco (Ed.), *Psychiatric Aspects of Organ Donation.* New York: Grune & Stratton, 1971.

Cattell, R. B., and Eber, W. E. *Handbook for the 16 Personality Factor Questionnaire.* Champaign, Ill.: Institute for Personality and Ability Testing, 1957.

Cohen, F., and Lazarus, R. S. "Active Coping Processes, Coping Dispositions, and Recovery from Surgery." *Psychosomatic Medicine,* 1973, *35,* 375–389.

Corday, E. "Status of Coronary Bypass Surgery." *Journal of the American Medical Association,* 1975, *231* (12), 1245–1247.

Dahlstrom, W. G., Welsh, G. S., and Dahlstrom, L. E. *An MMPI Handbook: A Guide to Use in Clinical Practice and Research.* (2 vols.) Minneapolis: University of Minnesota Press, 1975.

Danilowicz, D. A., and Gabriel, H. P. "Post-Cardiotomy Psychosis in Non-English Speaking Patients." *Psychiatry in Medicine,* 1971, *7,* 314–320.

Davis, J. M., and Casper, R. "Anti-Psychotic Drugs: Clinical Pharmacology and Therapeutic Use." *Drugs,* 1977, *14,* 260–282.

Dencker, S. J., and Sandahl, A. "Mental Disease After Operations for Mitral Stenosis." *Lancet,* 1961, *1,* 1230–1231.

Dencker, S. J., and Sandahl, A. "Major Mental Disturbances in a

Series of Patients Surgically Treated for Mitral Stenosis."
Acta Psychiatrica Scandinavica, 1962, *38,* 117–123.

Dietch, J. T. "Diagnosis of Organic Anxiety Disorders." *Psychosomatics,* 1981, *22* (8), 661–669.

Dubin, W. R., Field, H. R., and Gastfriend, D. R. "Postcardiotomy Delirium: A Critical Review." *Journal of Thoracic and Cardiovascular Surgery,* 1979, *77,* 586–594.

Edington, H. C. "Open-Heart Surgery: A Triple Threat." *Southern Medical Journal,* 1969, *61,* 160–166.

Egbert, L. D., and others. "Reduction of Post-Operative Pain by Encouragement and Instruction of Patients." *New England Journal of Medicine,* 1964, *270,* 825–827.

Egerton, N., and Kay, J. H. "Psychological Disturbances Associated with Open-Heart Surgery." *British Journal of Psychiatry,* 1964, *110,* 433–439.

Engel, G. L. "Psychogenic Pain and the Pain-Prone Patient." *American Journal of Medicine,* 1959, *26* (6), 899–918.

Engel, G. L. *Psychological Development in Health and Disease.* Philadelphia: Saunders, 1962.

Engel, G. L. "Conversion Symptoms." In C. M. MacBryde (Ed.), *Signs and Symptoms: Applied Physiology and Clinical Interpretation.* (5th ed.) Philadelphia: Lippincott, 1969.

Engel, G. L. "The Need for a New Medical Model: A Challenge for Biomedicine." *Science,* 1977, *196,* 129–136.

Engel, G. L. "A Life Setting Conducive to Illness: The Giving Up-Given Up Complex." *Bulletin of the Menninger Clinic,* 1980, *32,* 355–365.

Engel, G. L., and Romano, J. "Delirium: A Syndrome of Cerebral Insufficiency." *Journal of Chronic Diseases,* 1959, *9,* 260–277.

Engel, G. L., and Schmale, A. H., Jr. "Psychoanalytic Theory of Somatic Disorders: Conversion, Specificity, and the Disease Onset Situation." *Journal of the American Psychoanalytic Association,* 1967, *15,* 344–365.

Favalaro, R. G., and others. "Direct Myocardial Revascularization by Saphenous Vein Graft." *Annals of Thoracic Surgery,* 1970, *10,* 97–111.

Fiskind, E., and others. "Hypnoid Syndrome in Sensory Deprivation." In J. Wortis (Ed.), *Recent Advances in Biological Psychiatry.* Vol. 5. New York: Plenum, 1963.

Fox, H. M., Rizzo, N. D., and Gifford, S. "Psychological Observations of Patients Undergoing Mitral Surgery." *Psychosomatic Medicine,* 1954, *16,* 186-208.

Frank, K. A., Heller, S. S., and Kornfeld, D. S. "A Survey of Adjustment to Cardiac Surgery." *Archives of Internal Medicine,* 1972, *130,* 735-738.

Freyberger, H. "Psychotherapeutic Strategies in Patients Treated in Intensive Care Units." In H. Speidel and G. Rodewald (Eds), *Psychic and Neurological Dysfunctions After Open-Heart Surgery.* New York: Thieme-Stratton, 1978.

Freyhan, F. A., and others. "Psychiatric Complications Following Open-Heart Surgery." *Comprehensive Psychiatry,* 1971, *12,* 181-195.

Gilberstadt, H., and Sako, Y. "Intellectual and Personality Changes Following Open-Heart Surgery." *Archives of General Psychiatry,* 1967, *16,* 210-214.

Gilman, S. "Cerebral Disorders After Open-Heart Operations." *New England Journal of Medicine,* 1965, *272,* 489-498.

Goldstein, K. "On Emotions: Consideration from the Organismic Point of View." *Journal of Psychology,* 1951, *31,* 37-49.

Groves, J. E. "Management of the Borderline Patient on a Medical or Surgical Ward: The Psychiatric Consultant's Role." *International Journal of Psychiatry in Medicine,* 1975, *6,* 337-348.

Groves, J. E. "Taking Care of the Hateful Patient." *New England Journal of Medicine,* 1978, *298,* 883-887.

Gundle, M. J., and others. "Psychosocial Outcome After Coronary Artery Surgery." *American Journal of Psychiatry,* 1980, *137,* 1591-1594.

Hackett, T. P., and Cassem, N. H. (Eds.). *Massachusetts General Hospital Handbook of General Hospital Psychiatry.* St. Louis: Mosby, 1978.

Hazan, S. J. "Psychiatric Complications Following Cardiac Surgery. Part I: A Review Article." *Journal of Thoracic and Cardiovascular Surgery,* 1966a, *51,* 307-319.

Hazan, S. J. "Psychiatric Complications Following Cardiac Surgery. Part II: A Working Hypothesis—The Chemical Approach." *Journal of Thoracic and Cardiovascular Surgery,* 1966b, *51,* 320-325.

Healy, K. M. "Does Pre-Operative Instruction Make a Difference?" *American Journal of Nursing,* 1968, *68,* 62-67.

Heller, S. S., and others. "Psychiatric Complications of Open-Heart Surgery." *New England Journal of Medicine,* 1970, *283,* 1015-1020.

Heller, S. S., and others. "Psychological Outcome Following Open-Heart Surgery." *Archives of Internal Medicine,* 1974, *134,* 908-914.

Heller, S. S., and others. "Delirium After Coronary Artery Bypass Surgery." In H. Speidel and G. Rodewald (Eds.), *Psychic and Neurological Dysfunctions After Open-Heart Surgery.* New York: Thieme-Stratton, 1978.

Henn, F. A. "Complications of Antipsychotic Drug Therapy." *Resident and Staff Physician,* Feb. 1982, pp. 122-131.

Henrichs, T. F., MacKenzie, J. W., and Almond, C. H. "Psychological Adjustment and Acute Response to Open-Heart Surgery." *Journal of Nervous and Mental Disease,* 1969, *148,* 158-164.

Henrichs, T. F., MacKenzie, J. W., and Almond, C. H. "Psychological Adjustment and Psychiatric Complications Following Open-Heart Surgery." *Journal of Nervous and Mental Disease,* 1971, *152,* 332-345.

Henrichs, T. F., and Waters, W. F. "Psychological Adjustment and Response to Open-Heart Surgery: Some Methodological Considerations." *British Journal of Psychiatry,* 1972, *120,* 491-496.

Javid, H., and others. "Neurological Abnormalities Following Open-Heart Surgery." *Journal of Thoracic and Cardiovascular Surgery,* 1969, *58,* 502-509.

Jenkins, C. D., and others. "Coronary Artery Bypass Surgery: Physical, Psychological, Social, and Economic Outcomes Six Months Later." *Journal of the American Medical Association,* 1983, *250,* 782-788.

Kaplan, H. S. *The New Sex Therapy*. New York: Brunner/Mazel, 1974.

Kaplan, S. M. "Psychological Aspects of Cardiac Disease." *Psychosomatic Medicine*, 1956, *18*, 221-233.

Kasl, S. V., and Cobb, S. "Some Psychological Factors Associated with Illness Behavior and Selected Illnesses." *Journal of Chronic Diseases*, 1964, *17*, 325-330.

Kasl, S. V., and Cobb, S. "Health Behavior, Illness Behavior, and Sick Role Behavior." *Archives of Environmental Health*, 1966, *12*, 246-254.

Katz, J. Personal communication, 1978.

Kennedy, J. A., and Bakst, H. "The Influence of Emotions on the Outcome of Cardiac Surgery: A Predictive Study." *Bulletin of the New York Academy of Medicine*, 1966, *42*, 811-849.

Kimball, C. P. "Psychological Responses to the Experience of Open-Heart Surgery." *American Journal of Psychiatry*, 1969, *126*, 348-359.

Kimball, C. P. "The Experience of Open-Heart Surgery: Determinants of Post-Operative Behavior." *Psychotherapy and Psychosomatics*, 1970, *18*, 259-274.

Kimball, C. P. "The Experience of Open-Heart Surgery: Toward a Definition and Understanding of Postcardiotomy Delirium." *Archives of General Psychiatry*, 1972, *27*, 57-63.

Klein, R. F., and others. "Transfer from a Coronary Care Unit." *Archives of Internal Medicine*, 1968, *122*, 104-108.

Knox, S. J. "Severe Psychiatric Disturbances in the Post-Operative Period—A Five-Year Survey of Belfast Hospitals." *Journal of Mental Sciences*, 1961, *107*, 1078-1096.

Knox, S. J. "Psychiatric Aspects of Mitral Valvotomy." *British Journal of Psychiatry*, 1963, *109*, 656-668.

Kornfeld, D. S. "Psychiatric Complications of Cardiac Surgery." *International Psychiatry Clinics*, 1967, *4*, 115-131.

Kornfeld, D. S., Zimberg, S., and Malm, J. R. "Psychiatric Complications of Open-Heart Surgery." *New England Journal of Medicine*, 1965, *273*, 287-292.

Kornfeld, D. S., and others. "Personality and Psychological Factors in Postcardiotomy Delirium." *Archives of General Psychiatry*, 1974, *31*, 249-253.

Kornfeld, D. S., and others. "Delirium After Coronary Artery Bypass Surgery." *Journal of Cardiovascular Surgery,* 1978, *76,* 93-96.

Kraft, I. A. "Psychiatric Complications of Cardiac Transplantation." *Seminars in Psychiatry,* 1971, *3* (1), 58-69.

Layne, O. L., and Yudofsky, S. C. "Postoperative Psychosis in Cardiotomy Patients: The Role of Organic and Psychiatric Factors." *New England Journal of Medicine,* 1971, *284,* 518-520.

Lazarus, H. R., and Hagens, J. H. "Prevention of Psychosis Following Open-Heart Surgery." *American Journal of Psychiatry,* 1968, *124,* 1190-1195.

Lee, W. H., Jr., and others. "Effects of Extracorporeal Circulation on Personality and Cerebration." *Annals of Thoracic Surgery,* 1969, *7,* 562-570.

Lee, W. H., Jr., and others. "Effects of Extracorporeal Circulation upon Behavior, Personality, and Brain Function. Part II: Hemodynamics, Metabolic, and Psychometric Correlations." *Annals of Surgery,* 1971, *173,* 1013-1023.

Lev, M. "Congenital Heart Disease." In O. Saphir (Ed.), *A Text on Systemic Pathology.* Vol. 1. New York: Grune & Stratton, 1958.

Lindemann, E. "Symptomatology and Management of Acute Grief." *American Journal of Psychiatry,* 1944, *101,* 141-148.

Lipowski, A. J. "Delirium, Clouding of Consciousness and Confusion." *Journal of Nervous and Mental Disease,* 1967, *145,* 227-255.

Lucia, W., and McGuire, L. B. "Rehabilitation and Functional Status After Surgery for Valvular Heart Disease." *Archives of Internal Medicine,* 1970, *126,* 995-1000.

Lunde, D. "Psychiatric Complications of Heart Transplant." *American Journal of Psychiatry,* 1969, *126,* 369-373.

McKegney, F. P. "The Intensive Care Syndrome: The Definition, Treatment, and Prevention of a New 'Disease of Medical Progress.' " *Connecticut Medicine,* 1966, *30,* 633-636.

Marks, R. M., and Sachar, E. J. "Undertreatment of Medical Patients with Narcotic Analgesics." *Annals of Internal Medicine,* 1973, *78,* 173-181.

Menninger, K. A. "Polysurgery and Polysurgical Addiction." *Psychoanalytic Quarterly,* 1934, *3,* 173-199.

Meyer, B. C., Blacher, R. S., and Brown, F. "A Clinical Study of Psychiatric and Psychological Aspects of Mitral Surgery." *Psychosomatic Medicine,* 1961, *23,* 194-218.

Miller, L. J. "Informed Consent." *Journal of the American Medical Association,* 1980, *244* (18), 2100-2103.

Mumford, E., Schlesinger, H. J., and Glass, G. V. "The Effects of Psychological Intervention on Recovery from Surgery and Heart Attacks: An Analysis of the Literature." *American Journal of Public Health,* 1982, *72* (2), 141-152.

Nadelson, T. "The Psychiatrist in the Surgical Intensive Care Unit. I: Post-Operative Delirium." *Archives of Surgery,* 1976, *111,* 113-117.

Netter, F. H. *The Ciba Collection of Medical Illustrations.* Vol. 5. Summit, N.J.: Ciba Pharmaceutical Company, 1969.

Parsons, T., and Fox, R. "Illness, Therapy, and the Modern Urban American Family." *Journal of Social Issues,* 1952, *8,* 31-46.

Priest, W. S., and others. "The Neurologic, Psychiatric, and Psychologic Aspects of Cardiac Surgery." *Medical Clinics of North America,* Jan. 1957, pp. 155-169.

Rabiner, C. J., and Willner, A. E. "Psychopathology Observed on Follow-Up After Coronary Bypass Surgery." *Journal of Nervous and Mental Disease,* 1976, *163,* 295-301.

Rabiner, C. J., Willner, A. E., and Fishman, J. "Psychiatric Complications Following Coronary Bypass Surgery." *Journal of Nervous and Mental Disease,* 1975, *160,* 342-348.

Rubinstein, D., and Thomas, J. K. "Psychiatric Findings in Cardiotomy Patients." *American Journal of Psychiatry,* 1969, *126,* 360-369.

Shealy, A. E., and Walker, S. F. "MMPI Prediction of Intellectual Changes Following Cardiac Surgery." *Journal of Nervous and Mental Disease,* 1978, *166,* 263-267.

Silverstone, J. T., Tannahill, M. M., and Ireland, J. A. "Psychiatric Aspects of Profound Hypothermia in Open-Heart Surgery." *Journal of Thoracic and Cardiovascular Surgery,* 1970, *59,* 193-200.

Sime, A. M. "Relationship of Pre-Operative Fear, Type of Coping, and Information Received About Surgery to Recovery from Surgery." *Journal on Perspectives in Social Psychology,* 1976, *34,* 716-724.

Solomon, P., and others. "Sensory Deprivation." Symposium held at Harvard Medical School, Harvard University, Cambridge, Mass., 1961.

Sos, J., and Cassem, N. H. "The Intravenous Use of Haloperidol for Acute Delirium in Intensive Care Settings." In H. Speidel and G. Rodewald (Eds.), *Psychic and Neurological Dysfunctions After Open-Heart Surgery.* New York: Thieme-Stratton, 1978.

Surman, O. S., and others. "Usefulness of Psychiatric Intervention in Patients Undergoing Cardiac Surgery." *Archives of General Psychiatry,* 1974, *30,* 830-835.

Sveinnson, I. S. "Postoperative Psychosis After Heart Surgery." *Journal of Thoracic and Cardiovascular Surgery,* 1975, *70,* 717-726.

Symmes, J. C., Lenkei, C. M., and Berman, N. D. "Influence of Aortocoronary Bypass Surgery on Employment." *Canadian Medical Association Journal,* 1978, *118,* 268-270.

Tufo, H. M., Ostfeld, A. M., and Shekelle, R. "Central Nervous System Dysfunction Following Open-Heart Surgery." *Journal of the American Medical Association,* 1970, *212,* 1333-1340.

Weisman, A. D., and Hackett, T. P. "Psychosis After Eye Surgery." *New England Journal of Medicine,* 1958, *258,* 1284-1289.

Weiss, S. M. "Psychological Adjustment Following Open-Heart Surgery." *Journal of Nervous and Mental Disease,* 1966, *143,* 363-368.

West, L. J., and others. "Psychosis of Sleep Deprivation." *Annals of the New York Academy of Sciences,* 1962, *96,* 66-70.

Willner, A. E., and others. "Analogical Reasoning and Post-Operative Outcome in Patients Scheduled for Open-Heart Surgery." *Archives of General Psychiatry,* 1976, *33,* 255-259.

Wolpe, J., and Lazarus, A. A. *Behavior Therapy Techniques.* Elmsford, N.Y.: Pergamon Press, 1966.

Yalom, I. D. *Existential Psychotherapy.* New York: Basic Books, 1980.

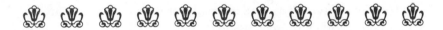

4

Coronary Artery Disease: Reducing Risk of Illness and Aiding Recovery

Andrew M. Razin, Ph.D., M.D.

Of the several cardiac problems considered in this volume, the one most commonly encountered in medical and psychotherapeutic practice, and the one that most broadly bears on other cardiac problems, is coronary artery disease (CAD). Hypertension, for example, derives a large part of its significance as a risk factor for CAD; arrhythmias often occur in the context of, or as a result of, CAD; and cardiac surgery is perhaps most commonly performed to correct the hemodynamic and electrical patho-

Sections of this chapter represent updates and modifications of previous publications (see Razin entries in list of references at the end of the chapter). I am deeply indebted to Carmen Correa and to Jessica Schairer, Charles Swencionis, Herbert Weiner, and Lenore Zohman for their valuable contributions to the clinical and research experiences that enabled me to write this chapter.

physiology associated with CAD. The centrality of CAD is still
further underlined by its severity. For many years CAD has
been the leading cause of death in this country in adults over
forty years of age. The full magnitude of this severity, moreover, is even greater when we consider the incidence and prevalence of nonfatal CAD events. And, while CAD incidence and
mortality have been declining over the last several years (presumably because of improved acute care facilities and increased
national attention to risk factor reduction), CAD has nonetheless retained its position as the leading cause of death.

What Is Coronary Artery Disease?

To discuss psychosocial interventions in CAD patients,
we must understand what CAD is. CAD is a broad, generic term,
including both atherosclerotic and nonatherosclerotic disease of
the coronary arteries, as well as resultant disease of the heart itself. Like all other muscle tissue, the myocardium (the muscle
that comprises virtually all of the functioning pumping heart)
requires oxygen, in amounts that vary with the effort (rate and
contractile force) with which the heart is pumping. The coronary arteries (which take their name from the crown-shaped ar-
rangement that they form around the upper portion of the
heart) branch out to provide the heart itself with oxygenated
blood. When the supply of oxygen is insufficient for the mo-
mentary level of demand, ischemia is said to occur. Often,
though not always, such ischemia is experienced as chest pain.
When the ischemia is sufficiently prolonged or severe, myocardial tissue dies (infarcts), and the patient is said to have suffered
a myocardial infarction or heart attack. The amount and location of infarcted tissue determine the severity of the myocardial
infarction (MI). A massive MI, involving large portions of the left
ventricle (the primary pumping chamber for the entire body),
may kill its victim, while a mild MI, involving only a small area
of (hemodynamically and electrically) less significant tissue,
might leave its victim able to resume a fully active, long life. Because the conductive (electrical) activity of the heart typically
changes in characteristic ways during and after MI, electrocardi-

ograms (ECGs) will usually be diagnostic. In addition, with the death of muscle tissue, certain enzymes are liberated from within muscle cells to the bloodstream; these "cardiac enzymes" will therefore appear in increased concentration in the blood, and such elevations are also diagnostic of MI.

There are several reasons for which the coronary arteries may not permit sufficient flow of blood. Most commonly, as we age, lipids such as cholesterol deposit themselves as placques (or atheromata) on the inner walls of these and other arteries, progressively reducing the inner cross-sectional area (lumen) of the artery and thus reducing blood flow. In addition to reducing luminal size, these placques also eventually "harden" the arteries; that is, they reduce the arteries' elastic ability to distend on demand, in order to allow increased blood flow. This hardening process is called arteriosclerosis or atherosclerosis and is accepted as the most common cause of CAD and MI. Additionally, a blood clot, or thrombus, may form in, or find its way into, the coronary arteries. Either alone or, more especially, in combination with atherosclerosis, such a clot may occlude an artery or its branches, forming a coronary occlusion or thrombosis, which term has often loosely been used synonymously with MI. Finally, the rings of smooth muscle, which comprise a significant part of the coronary artery walls, may spasm, thereby constricting the arteries and reducing blood flow. Thus, coronary spasm may—alone or in combination with the above mechanisms—also cause ischemia. There are additional, less common causes of coronary artery insufficiency, which are well described in the cardiology text of Hurst, Logue, and Walter (1978).

If the ischemia remits promptly enough, no permanent myocardial damage results, although the victim typically feels transient chest pain. Such transient, noninfarcting ischemia caused by atherosclerosis is recognized as angina pectoris—a characteristic syndrome of chest pain, usually precipitated by physical exertion and/or psychological stress and relieved by rest and/or medications that dilate the coronary arteries (for example, nitroglycerin). Angina resulting from arterial spasm is designated Prinzmetal's, or atypical, angina. Patients may have angina that remains stable and possibly never worsens to become a frank MI, or they may have progressively worsening "crescendo" angina, or they may suffer MI without any antecedent angina, or they may suffer a "silent" (asymptomatic) MI that is recognized only subsequently. Finally, patients, with or without documented CAD, may display "pseudoangina"—that is, pain in some ways resembling angina pectoris but not of ischemic etiology. CAD is thus a very heterogeneous group of phenomena etiologically, prognostically, and phenomenologically.

Over the past several decades, literally dozens of factors—physiological, anatomical, behavioral, social, metabolic—have been proposed as CAD risk factors. Of these, a handful have been found by careful research to contribute in some causative way to increased CAD risk. Hypertension, cigarette smoking, and serum cholesterol levels seem to be "the big three" in magnitude of risk increase; sex, age, family history of CAD, presence of diabetes mellitus, sedentary lifestyle, and obesity pose additional risk.

Psychosocial Factors and Sequelae

For many centuries both practicing physicians and laypeople have believed that, in addition to the "biological" risk factors, a variety of psychological factors—such as "stress," anxiety, and depression—could also predispose to or precipitate CAD events. But until the 1960s there was very little rigorously derived empirical evidence to support this widespread belief. Since that time research evidence of acceptable quality has clearly indicated associations, some of which appear to be causal, between several psychosocial factors and CAD. An examination of the excellent reviews by Jenkins (1971, 1976) and others (Blackburn, 1974; Russek and Russek, 1976; Roskies, 1980) yields the following conclusions concerning these associations:

1. There are definite positive associations *of some kind* between several psychosocial factors and CAD development.
2. The strength of these associations, however, varies across different psychosocial factors. Thus, life-stress events, anxiety, depression, and Type A behavior show relatively consistent associations, while demographic indicators, socio-

economic status, socioeconomic mobility, and socioeconomic incongruity show weak or inconsistent associations. The Type A Behavior Pattern (TABP) has clearly been the single most extensively studied psychosocial factor, and probably the one most strongly associated with CAD. In our view, research on the TABP over the past two decades has been largely responsible for the increased interest in and acceptance of psychosocial CAD risk factors.

3. The specificity of the above associations varies. Life-stress events and neuroticism, for example, seem linked to general morbidity, while anxiety, depression, and life dissatisfaction may be more specifically linked to angina.

4. The precise causal nature or mechanisms of these associations have not been clearly demonstrated, even among the strongest of these associations.

5. The highly complex interplay of social, economic, cultural, psychosocial, psychobiological, genetic, physiological, endocrinological, and other factors will undoubtedly continue to make research in this area extraordinarily difficult.

6. A definitive understanding of the relationships between psychosocial factors and CAD development, although brought closer by recent research, still eludes us.

With the heterogeneity of prognoses and severity described above, it should not be surprising that the psychosocial sequelae, or impacts, of CAD are also quite variable, and it would thus be futile and misleading to attempt to characterize CAD's impact in any single way. By focusing specifically on MI, however, we can delineate factors that are associated with differential short- and long-term patient reactions. Our own clinical experience and the existent literature on post-MI recovery (well reviewed by Croog, Levine, and Lurie, 1968, and by Doehrman, 1977) provide us with the following conclusions:

1. Above and beyond the temporary disruptive psychosocial functioning that one would expect with acute CAD, one finds long-lasting emotional distress, family turmoil, and occupational problems in a significant minority (perhaps 25 percent) of patients.

2. Coronary care unit (CCU) patients typically do *not* experience short- or long-term emotional disturbance as a result of CCU events and procedures (such as witnessing cardiac arrests or being connected to cardiac monitors).

3. Emotional distress, particularly depression, tends to peak *after* hospital discharge. Family tensions are common during convalescence. Patients seek and receive most of their social support from relatives, friends, and their doctors rather than from formal institutional or professional services.

4. As one might expect, occupational adjustment problems are greater among blue-collar workers, less educated patients, those with lasting emotional distress, and those with more serious medical problems.

5. Most patients do *not* return to previous levels of sexual activity; this failure is due more often to reported psychological concerns than to "physical" consequences of their illness.

6. Higher socioeconomic status (SES) and marital stability seem to be associated with good prognosis. The long-term psychological and physiological benefits of physical exercise, despite broad endorsement, have not been well demonstrated and actually remain controversial among some physicians.

7. The short- and long-term importance of denial is intriguing though unclear. A significant proportion of patients tend to minimize or even totally deny the occurrence or affective significance of their MI. There is some evidence that those who do so in the acute and immediate postacute phases may fare better prognostically than nondeniers. Over the longer run, though, this association is less clear. Multiple methodological problems preclude clear conclusions on this issue.

8. At the other end of the spectrum of reactions, unwarranted "cardiac invalidism" seems to be a common, and frequently refractory, problem once it develops, but it may be preventable by appropriate, *early* psychosocial and medical interventions.

Psychosocial Interventions

There are several generally thoughtful and astute reviews of this literature. Two of these (Doehrman, 1977; Frank, Heller, and Kornfeld, 1979) focus primarily on recovery; another (Blanchard and Miller, 1977) examines several cardiovascular diseases and pays only limited attention to CAD; still another (Thoresen, Telch, and Eagleston, 1981) focuses exclusively on Type A behavior. Another covers both uncontrolled and controlled studies of MI, angina, and "cardiac neurosis" (Razin, 1982). Finally, interventions aimed at reduction of traditional "biological" or "psychobiological" risk factors—such as obesity, hyperlipidemias, smoking, and physical inactivity—have been the focus of two additional reviews (Kasl, 1975; McAlister and others, 1976). Here, since our focus is primarily on treatment rather than research methodology, we shall present in summary form the conclusions of these reviews and encourage the reader interested in methodological issues or greater detail to consult the reviews themselves. We have organized the literature into three sections: *prevention,* which considers primary and secondary CAD-prevention efforts; *acute-phase intervention,* focusing on interventions during coronary care unit confinement; and *convalescent/rehabilitation-phase intervention,* covering the post-CCU hospitalization period and subsequent (postdischarge) period.

Prevention

Attempts at primary and secondary prevention of CAD have generally focused on reducing one or more of the known "risk factors": elevated serum cholesterol, hypertension, cigarette smoking, diabetes mellitus, and lack of exercise. With the important exceptions of smoking and hypertension, however, there has been disappointingly meager evidence that reduction of these factors actually prevents CAD (Rosenman, 1978). As indicated above, several psychosocial factors have gained credibility as "risk factors" over the past two decades. Some of these risk factors, such as neuroticism or delay in seeking medical

attention, *could,* in our current state of knowledge and methodological sophistication, be assessed for CAD-preventive effects.
To date, however, only one has been the focus of prevention research: the Type A behavior pattern. Review of the preventive
intervention literature is thus confined to it.

   TABP: Definition and Association with CAD. According
to Rosenman and Friedman, who originally identified it, the
Type A behavior pattern is "a characteristic action-emotion
complex which is exhibited by those individuals who are en-
gaged in a relatively chronic struggle to obtain an unlimited
number of poorly defined things from their environment in
the shortest period of time and, if necessary, against the oppos-
ing efforts of other things or persons in this same environment"
(Friedman, 1969, p. 84). It is "an overt behavior syndrome or
style of living characterized by extremes of competitiveness,
striving for achievement, aggressiveness (sometimes stringently
repressed), haste, impatience, restlessness, hyperalertness, ex-
plosiveness of speech, tenseness of facial musculature, and feelings of being under the pressure of time and under the challenge of responsibility. Persons having this pattern are often so
deeply committed to their vocation or profession that other
aspects of their lives are relatively neglected. Not all aspects of
this syndrome or pattern need be present for a person to be
classified as possessing it. The pattern is neither a personality
trait nor a standard reaction to a challenging situation, but
rather the reaction of a characterologically predisposed person
to a situation which challenges him. Different kinds of situations evoke maximal reactions from different persons" (Jenkins,
1971, p. 244).

      Furthermore, one can assess the pattern in some detail by
noting the characteristic values, style of thought, interpersonal
relationships, style of response, gestures and movements, facial
expressions, and breathing patterns observed in interview, self-
report questionnaire, and/or voice recordings (Jenkins, 1975).

      The TABP is not identical with anxiety (actually, Type A
individuals are described as relatively free of anxiety), or with
"stress," a term usually used to refer to certain noxious stimuli
and situations or to the reactions (for instance, alarm, discom-

fort, pain, or characteristic physiological changes) to such stimuli. The TABP, then, is neither the stressor nor the stress response but, rather, a style of behavior with which some people respond to challenging situations.

Much remains problematic about the Type A pattern. We still do not know, for example, whether Type A behavior is identical with "true" coronary-prone behavior or how it is related to stress; there are also problems with measurement, meaning, and specificity. Nonetheless, the basic conclusion seems relatively sound and incontrovertible: Whatever the association with other risk factors (such as serum cholesterol levels, smoking, and hypertension), the Type A pattern does seem to be clearly and independently associated with increased CAD risk. This has been shown prospectively in the eight-and-a-half-year Western Collaborative Group study of multiple risk factors (Rosenman and others, 1975), the Framingham study (Haynes and others, 1978), and at least seven smaller prospective studies, as well as twelve retrospective studies in the past decade alone (Jenkins, 1976). The relationship has not been proven to be causal, though, and it does not account for a major proportion of the variance in predicting new CAD. But the relationship does clearly seem to exist: Type A men under fifty (and perhaps under sixty) have about twice the CAD risk of Type Bs; their risk of recurrent myocardial infarction or fatal myocardial infarction is at least as elevated. Furthermore, arteriography and autopsy studies tend to confirm correlations between degree of atherosclerosis and the presence of the TABP (Jenkins, 1975).

The reader interested in broader critical considerations of the many other issues in TABP research (TABP-CAD associations among various demographic groups, psychological correlates of the TABP, measurement problems) should consult the general reviews (Roskies, 1980; Dembroski and others, 1980; Cooper, Detre, and Weiss, 1978; Rosenman and Chesney, 1980). Consideration of some pathophysiological correlates of the TABP (such as increased red blood cell sludging and increased catecholamine response to stress) can be found in Friedman (1977) and in Rosenman and Chesney (1980).

TABP: Modifying the Behavior. As the TABP became increasingly known and its credibility as a risk factor more widely accepted, reports of attempted modification of TABP began to appear about eight years ago. Detailed critical descriptions of these reports (published before 1982) are available (Razin, 1982, 1984d). Nearly all of these (nine) systematic and (three) nonsystematic studies show "positive" outcome of one kind or another, and nearly all suggest relatively specific diminution of at least some aspect(s) of the Type A pattern. At this stage, however, these findings should be considered no more than promising. In addition to multiple methodological limitations, there are only modest data on durability, virtually no data on generalizability, and absolutely no data on CAD risk reduction value of any of these improvements.

Quite significantly, however, two more recent studies strengthen this promising picture. In the first, Friedman and his associates (1982) have provided a preliminary report on the only large-scale longitudinal study of TABP reduction, and the impact of such reduction on subsequent CAD. They randomly assigned 900 post-MI patients to either traditional-risk-factor-oriented cardiological counseling groups ($N = 300$) or to groups that, in addition, provided a variety of didactic and cognitive-behavioral techniques aimed at TABP reduction ($N = 600$). An additional 135 subjects volunteered to serve as no-counseling controls. After the first of five years, the rates of reinfarction and cardiovascular death were markedly lower among TABP-counseled subjects than among untreated controls, and the rate of nonfatal infarction was lower among TABP-counseled subjects than among cardiological-counseled-only subjects and among untreated controls.

In the well-controlled second study, Levenkron and associates (1983) found that a similar behavioral program (and, to a nearly equivalent extent, a supportive group intervention) seemed to lower stress-induced serum free fatty acid elevations. Thus, on two crucial issues—the reducibility of physiological hyperreactivity and the reducibility of CAD risks via TABP reduction—promising evidence has been adduced.

There nonetheless remain additional problems in TABP

reduction. First, we have not yet demonstrated which of the several components that comprise the multidimensional TABP are truly CAD pathogenic. Nor have we completely identified those non-TABP behaviors that are CAD pathogenic (truly coronary prone). Thus, as long as these distinctions between the TABP and true coronary-prone behavior remain unclear, we cannot be precise about which TABP behaviors to target therapeutically. There is, to be sure, suggestive evidence that only competitive drive, impatience, and hostility are pathogenic (Matthews and others, 1977) and therefore that job involvement and other TABP components may be incidental, but such suggestions have not yet been corroborated, nor have they been studied systematically.

Second, while Type A status doubles the risk of new CAD in a vulnerable population, only 1 percent of Type A subjects develop CAD per year (Rosenman and others, 1975). Furthermore, 50–75 percent of asymptomatic at-risk males would be classified by current assessment techniques as Type A. Thus, there remain problems of specificity and measurement selection (for example, interview versus self-report) and refinement. When we add to these problems the likely resistance of the manifestly "healthy" at-risk population, *and* of their frequently Type A physicians, it seems premature at this early stage to recommend large-scale TABP-reducing primary CAD-prevention projects. While even a proportionally small reduction of CAD incidence (such as 5 percent) would entail 50,000 fewer MIs per year, we must become more precise in specifying, assessing, and treating the pathogenic (truly coronary-prone) aspects of the TABP before embarking on such massive campaigns. At this point, then, more limited, secondary-preventive efforts, aimed at those already stricken with CAD (and thus "proven" to be truly coronary prone), should be more feasible and more heuristic (even though, with this diseased population, the degree to which existent anatomical pathology and pathophysiology can be arrested or reversed poses another set of problems).

Finally, TABP-modification research has not yet advanced to the point of addressing the very likely wide physiological heterogeneity within the large group of people currently classified as Type A. Given the ubiquity and the psychological heterogeneity of Type A individuals, it seems unlikely that we shall find a single uniform physiology, or physiological response to TABP modification, among these individuals. It therefore becomes crucial for intervention research to tap concurrent self-report, behavioral, and physiological data channels for meaningful outcome assessment.

Acute-Phase Intervention

There have been very few systematic studies of intervention during the acute phase. There is, however, a fair-sized anecdotal and exhortatory-prescriptive literature, summarized by Doehrman (1977), based on the psychiatric liaison-consultation experiences of several clinicians in coronary care units (CCUs), and there are a few more systematic studies describing patients' reactions to CCUs.

Patient Reactions During the Acute Phase. Most reports indicate that patients are generally reassured by the CCU, particularly by the visible presence of equipment (Hackett, Cassem, and Wishnie, 1968; Lenzner and Aronson, 1972), and of other patients (Dominian and Dobson, 1969; Leigh and others, 1972), in "open" CCUs. On the other hand, there is psychological (Dominian and Dobson, 1969) and physiological (Bruhn and others, 1970) evidence that a significant proportion (33-62 percent, depending on defining criteria) of MI patients experience at least some degree of distress, which may be denied or suppressed. Cassem and Hackett (1971) have developed a model for the time course of such distress (based on the timing and nature of requests for psychiatric consultation). According to the model, anxiety predominates on post-MI days 1 and 2 and subsequently declines, depression peaks on days 3-5 as the impact of the MI is felt, denial may predominate early (on day 2) to defend against these intense feelings, and chronic character traits occur later (days 4-6). Subsequent reports have tended to confirm the ubiquity and time course for anxiety, as well as the ubiquity of the other affective-behavioral reactions, but the time courses for these latter reactions have not been confirmed (Doehrman, 1977).

More extreme reactions—such as altered states of consciousness, psychotic episodes, and deliria—have, of course, also been widely reported. And there has been controversy concerning the etiology of such states, with postsurgical metabolic imbalances, medication effects, cardiogenic hypoxia, and intensive care unit environments all being suspect. There nonetheless seems to be a degree of consensus that psychosocial factors play at least some etiological role, most likely in interaction with metabolic conditions. Kornfeld, Zimberg, and Malm (1965) and Kimball (1978), for example, emphasize the importance of the uniquely strange intensive care environments, which provide both overstimulation and understimulation, lack familiar figures, and often minimize communication and environmental cues of diurnal sequence. As the findings of Leigh and his associates (1972) and others suggest, amelioration of these environmental anomalies may lessen the intensity and perhaps the frequency of major psychiatric disturbance. Chapter Three in this volume provides a comprehensive discussion of these issues.

In a series of studies, Lynch and his associates (Lynch and others, 1974; Mills and others, 1976) have demonstrated the susceptibility of cardiac arrhythmias in CAD and other CCU patients to a variety of "socioclinical" CCU events (such as staff or family visits and departures, pulse palpation, or central venous pressure (CVP) recordings). While specific intervention recommendations do not emerge readily from this work, what does emerge is the exquisite sensitivity of the compromised heart (and, as the authors point out, the intact heart) to psychosocial stimuli. This sensitivity, however, need not portend only danger. Arrhythmia patients found to be particularly sensitive to socioclinical events might be those most easily taught (via such techniques as biofeedback and relaxation) to control arrhythmias.

Denial During the Acute Phase. Most observers of acute-phase coronary patients find denial to be ubiquitous. Hackett, Cassem, and Wishnie (1968), for example, found it so widespread that they were able to subclassify fifty CAD patients as "major" deniers (who reported no fear at all), "partial" deniers (who eventually acknowledged some fear), or "minimal" deniers (who readily acknowledged fear). They recommend use of this classification scheme for differential patient management planning. They also report that, while denial showed no relationship to predominant mood, deniers did tend to respond more positively to the ECG monitors. Other studies have found denial associated with less anxiety (Doehrman, 1977) and lower mortality (Roskies, 1980; Hackett, Cassem, and Wishnie, 1968), though the studies on mortality had insufficient subjects for appropriate statistical analysis.

While there are also reports questioning the apparent ubiquity or protective functionality of denial, the interstudy discrepancies seem in part to be due to the inconsistency and ambiguity with which the term is used. Usages of the term range from the conscious refusal to acknowledge verbally the occurrence of an MI, through various types of noncompliant behavior (presumably motivated by the wish to deny the illness), through repression or suppression of dysphoric affects, to the grossly delusional or hallucinatory loss of reality testing. It seems very unlikely that all these varied phenomena have identical functions and effects. Clearly, a broadly acceptable, reliable system of defining and classifying denial both quantitatively and qualitatively is needed. Hackett and Cassem (1974) have developed a denial rating scale, which represents a first step toward precision in this area, but to date the scale has not been widely used.

We might gain further understanding of the functions and effects of denial by considering the phase during which it occurs and how long it persists; a distinction may need to be drawn between those who (more adaptively?) deny only during the acute phase and those who deny more chronically. Thus, two uncontrolled reports (Soloff, 1978; Bartle and Bishop, 1974) suggest *greater* morbidity and mortality among chronic postacute deniers.

Effects of Transfer from CCU. Several studies (Hackett, Cassem, and Wishnie, 1968; Dominian and Dobson, 1969; Klein and others, 1968; Rahe, 1975) have noted adverse effects (increased depression, anxiety, reinfarction, arrhythmia, and serum cholesterol and uric acid levels) associated with transfer to general medical wards. In the one partially controlled intervention study of this phenomenon, Klein and his associates (1968) found fewer of these changes among patients who were systematically prepared for transfer and who were each followed throughout and after hospitalization by a single designated nurse and a single designated physician.

Guidelines for Acute-Phase Intervention. In addition to the recommendations that appear implicitly or explicitly in the above discussion, several other clinical guidelines emerge from the acute-phase literature. As with the above recommendations, these guidelines emerge from clinical experiences, and virtually none of them enjoys rigorously derived empirical supporting data. (1) Appropriate, well-timed, psychological intervention in the acute phase is beneficial and therefore should be *routinely* offered. (2) Intervention should be didactic, detailed, and repetitive. (3) Clinicians should take an open, honest approach to patients, showing compassion, confidence, and forthrightness. (4) Clinicians should be aware of the relative phasic specificity of patient reactions. (5) Anxiety should be treated supportively and thus minimized whenever possible. (6) Early physical mobilization should be encouraged.

Convalescent/Rehabilitative-Phase Interventions

There is a fairly substantial literature on this phase, though much of it is clinically based prescription, rather than systematic research. We shall present the guidelines that emerge concerning intervention in "routine" post-MI situations, and also intervention in "cardiac neurosis" and in anginoid syndromes.

"Routine" Post-MI Intervention. The literature and our own experience suggest the following guidelines for consulting or treating psychotherapists:

1. Intervention must be early. Nearly all clinicians (Soloff, 1978; Cassem and Hackett, 1973, 1977; Granger, 1974; Nagle, Gangola, and Picton-Robinson, 1971) stress the preventability of much convalescent-phase psychological distress, in-

validism, and recurrence of coronary events. Rehabilitative interventions, including physical mobilization, are recommended to begin *before* the patient leaves the CCU (Soloff, 1978; Cassem and Hackett, 1977), although lasting psychological benefit from early versus later physical mobilization has been difficult to demonstrate (Groden, Allison, and Shaw, 1967; Groden and Brown, 1970).

2. Intervention must be specific, systematic, graduated, and educative. Given that patient *perceptions* of their own health may be more important than actual clinical severity of MI in determining morale and return to work (Garrity, 1973a, 1973b), that these perceptions may bear little relationship to actual severity, that simple ignorance may prevent return to work (Nagle, Gangola, and Picton-Robinson, 1971), and that patients may respond adversely to unintended, nonverbal, or symbolic meanings of physicians' communications (Garrity, 1973b), it is not surprising that nearly all clinicians decry the vagueness or total absence of many physicians' explanations of CAD and rehabilitative plans. Beyond this, several clinicians (Garrity, 1973b; Wishnie, Hackett, and Cassem, 1971) recommend actively eliciting patients' fears and (mis-)conceptions (to prevent later destructive effects) and teaching patients that their behavior may affect their CAD (Cassem and Hackett, 1973; Granger, 1974; Wynn, 1967; Wishnie, Hackett, and Cassem, 1971).

3. Specific attention should be paid to depression. Post-MI depression seems remarkably ubiquitous both across patients and over time, perhaps up to three years post-MI (Verwoerdt and Dovenmuhle, 1964). Thus, physicians are urged to recognize it (in its varied manifestations and times of occurrences) and to treat it (Wynn, 1967), even as early as day 3 (Cassem and Hackett, 1973). In such early treatment, the physician should explicitly predict that the patient may well go through a temporary period of depression. This anticipation should legitimate (the communication of) such depression as part of the expectable course of recovery and should thus prevent the depression from "snowballing."

4. Social supports must be involved and mobilized. Again, there is near unanimity (Croog, Levine, and Lurie, 1968;

Thompson, 1977; Klein and others, 1968; Cassem and Hackett, 1973) that rehabilitative success in large part hinges on family, particularly spouse, education and involvement. Discouraging spouses from "walking on eggs" and helping families adopt realistic role changes are generally recommended.

Beyond these recommendations there is substantial, if indirect and poorly understood, evidence of the dangers of discharging post-MI patients to live alone. Whether by virtue of being married, remarried, or even owning a pet, those who live accompanied seem to enjoy lower cardiovascular mortality (Croog, Levine, and Lurie, 1968; Doehrman, 1977; Lynch, 1977; Helsing, Szklo, and Comstock, 1981). It thus seems reasonable that clinicians should exert efforts to reinforce family cohesiveness or generate new sources of companionship or support (for example, friends, extended family, "coronary clubs," pets).

5. Continuity and follow-up are essential. Several uncontrolled studies suggest that improvements in rehospitalization rates (Prince and Miranda, 1977), return to work (McGrath and Robinson, 1973), and other aspects of rehabilitation (Granger, 1974) are associated with programs providing medical staff continuity and follow-up.

In addition to the largely prescriptive, nonsystematic literature from which the above guidelines emerge, there are at least two additional anecdotal reports (Cathey and others, 1962; Stein, Murdaugh, and MacLeod, 1969) and four systematic studies (Thockloth and others, 1973; Gruen, 1975; Naismith and others, 1979; Baile and Engel, 1978) of individual therapy, as well as six uncontrolled reports (Mone, 1970; Bilodeau and Hackett, 1971; Weiner, Akabas, and Sommer, 1973; Golden, cited by Hackett, 1978; Frank, Heller, and Kornfeld, 1979; Soloff, 1979) and six controlled studies (Adsett and Bruhn, 1968; Ibrahim and others, 1974; Rahe and others, 1973, 1975, 1979; Roskies and others, 1978; Jenni and Wollersheim, 1979; Friedman and others, 1982) of group interventions. Since these studies are critically reviewed in detail elsewhere (Hackett, 1978; Frank, Heller, and Kornfeld, 1979; Razin, 1982, 1984a), we shall present here only summary comments on them.

The studies of individual therapy indicate that, while

nearly all report generally positive outcomes, there are serious methodological and/or reporting problems. Most studies lack controls or are purely anecdotal, "treatment" is often not defined, the positive outcome data are often of debatable clinical significance, and some data are internally inconsistent. Thus, the *suggestion* of favorable impact is made, but the clear clinical, particularly physiological, significance of individual post-MI psychotherapy remains to be demonstrated in a methodologically sound manner. Furthermore, although the types of therapy that seem successful are nonexploratory (that is, they are didactic, behavioral, and reality oriented), there are no definitive comparative data on which to base this conclusion.

Review of the studies of group therapy yields several conclusions. First, such treatment seems beneficial; there are moderate, consistent psychological gains and less consistent but clinically significant physiological CAD-prognostic gains from such treatment. Second, most of the studies to date—even the controlled studies—have major methodological problems. In particular, both psychological and physiological outcome criteria are questionable, and patient characteristics are unclearly specified. Well-specified, well-chosen self-report, behavioral, and correlative physiological data should be gathered at pre- and post-treatment and at follow-up. In addition, given the global impression of beneficial influence, much more refined, specific hypotheses must be formulated and tested. Thus, for example, there is not a single study comparing group and individual therapies for CAD patients, although clinical experience suggests that group therapy may have several advantages (Razin, 1984a). Furthermore, other issues—such as patient selection criteria, the timing and duration of treatment, the manner of spouse involvement, and the comparative efficacy of alternate treatments (for example family or self-control/behavioral)—are still unresolved. A few of the Type A behavior reduction studies—specifically those of Friedman and associates (1982) and Levenkron and associates (1983)—stand as notable exceptions to these methodological problems.

Intervention in Cardiac Neurosis/Cardiac Invalidism. These terms (and a variety of additional synonyms, such as neurocirculatory asthenia) have been applied somewhat interchangeably to either of two patient types: a younger, CAD-free group for whom the term designates a variant of anxiety neurosis with cardiac symptoms (palpitations, chest pain, tachycardia); and an older, CAD-ridden, symptomatically similar group whose dysfunction and dysphoria exceed medical warrant. Post-MI cardiac invalidism is common, found in as many as 50 percent of post-MI patients (Wynn, 1967); exceedingly costly; and troublesome to patients, their families, and their physicians.

Treatment of this neurosis/invalidism, however, is described solely in prescriptive reports emphasizing prevention. There are uncontrolled anecdotal reports of supportive psychodynamic therapy (Stein, Murdaugh, and MacLeod, 1969) and of behavioral intervention (Baile and Engel, 1978; Wickramasekera, 1974; Rifkin, 1968) and a "comparative study" of psychotherapy versus routine medical care and reassurance, in which the patients were anxiety neurotics and not specifically cardiac neurotics (Wheeler and others, 1950). The generally positive results in these reports should be seen as merely suggestive. Systematic controlled study of these costly and disabling syndromes, with carefully specified patient criteria, is clearly needed.

Intervention in Anginoid Syndromes. Closely related to cardiac neurosis/invalidism are the problems of "true" angina pectoris and pseudoangina ("angina innocens"). Angina is a very common and usually frightening symptom. Furthermore, it is often difficult to distinguish from pseudoangina (angina-like pain of nonischemic, usually noncardiac, origin), as White and associates (1955) and Garner and Falk (1970) indicate. Pseudoangina may be part of a cardiac invalidism.

The few intervention studies in this area are uncontrolled or unclearly reported (see the reviews by Razin, 1982, 1984b). With so little research, we have relied heavily on our own and other clinicians' experiences in formulating the following clinical guidelines for working with anginoid pain. Until systematic research assesses the utility of these interventions, the reader should keep in mind the limitations inherent in any such clinically based set of guidelines.

The consulting or treating psychotherapist should begin by thoroughly familiarizing himself with what is known medically about the patient and his anginoid pain. The therapist should, for example, be clear about the medical distinctions between angina and pseudoangina (see Razin, 1984c) and the degree of certainty attached to such criteria. Does the patient clearly manifest typical angina pectoris? Are his symptoms atypical in some way? What is the patient's overall medical status? Is CAD documented, suspected, or doubtful? What is its severity and prognosis? Is there a noncardiac medical/surgical history or condition? Much of this information may have to come from the primary physician or cardiologist, but the patient's understanding of these issues is also crucial for several reasons, including the significance of discrepancies between the physician's and the patient's understanding of his diagnosis, symptoms, and etiology. As several clinicians (for example, Hackett, 1978) point out, problematic (often psychogenic) pain syndromes often have at least some of their origin or exacerbation in the primary doctor–patient relationship.

The psychotherapist should complete a detailed "pain inquiry" as he would with any other pain patient (see Hackett, 1978). This inquiry should assess the quality, location, timing, and severity of the anginoid pain; the time and manner of its onset; the various treatments already attempted, including detailed information about medication, compliance, and side effects; and the patient's view of his primary physician. In addition, the physiological and psychological circumstances surrounding both short- and long-term fluctuations in the frequency and intensity of pain episodes—that is, immediate exertional, "emotional," or other precipitants, as well as longer-term (seasonal and life-change) conditions—should be assessed. Though we may deliberately avoid an interpretive stance with many anginoid patients, we wish for our own understanding to consider not only the possible psychogenic *etiology* of the pain but also its psychological *meaning*: Whatever its source, what is its psychological *impact* on the patient? The meaning of pain will in part determine pain-related behavior and thus must be sought if one is to design any pain management strategies. This meaning is, in turn, determined by several factors, including the symbolic and/or realistic significance attached to the heart; previous experience with CAD, other illness, or other pain; the patient's family's experiences with pain and heart disease; and cultural and socioeconomic norms regarding pain, pain behavior, and the heart. Thus, for example, since angina pectoris seems to be associated with greater socioeconomic mobility, relief from obligation of work and achievement may be a significant source of secondary gain for high-achieving patients.

Other guidelines that emerge from work with noncardiac chronic pain have relevance here as well. Psychotherapists, for example, are frequently asked to distinguish "functional" from "organic" pain. In practice, relatively few cases of chronic pain are so categorically distinguishable; very little chronic pain occurs without at least some contribution from both psyche and soma. Such pain, except in cases of malingering, is always "real" because, regardless of etiology, the patient *feels* is. No matter how sophisticated the technology we might employ, a subjective experience such as pain is—in principle, and not only in practice—*not* reducible to objective data. We must remember, moreover, that pseudoangina often occurs in patients with documented angina pectoris. Thus, the therapist should not, either explicitly or implicitly, refer to the pain as imaginary. Nor should he gloss over the patient's experience of it; on the contrary, he should spend a great deal of time focusing on the pain, both to gather data diagnostically and to convey a genuine interest in, and valuation of, the patient's subjective experience —an interest the patient often perceives as lacking in his other medical relationships.

The physiology of pain changes with duration, such that, after six months, the afferent and efferent nociceptive pathways involved may change, thus providing a meaningful basis for the distinction between acute and chronic pain. In practice the psychotherapist's involvement is often not sought until the pain has become chronic. This lateness tends to make therapeutic work more difficult: The patient is more likely to have undergone coronary angiography and even bypass surgery, which, if it produces little relief, may entrench the patient's sense of failure, worthlessness, anger at doctors, and other such feelings. Furthermore, his physicians are more likely to view him as a "crock" or malingerer. Thus, a career as a medical misfit may have begun. *Timely* psychotherapeutic intervention, then, is crucial. And, while it may be difficult to detect psychogenic components in the early stages of pain, there are some guideposts: history of polysurgery, and/or multiple physician changes, and/or multiple, vague, or atypical organ system involvement; personal identity based largely on being "sickly"; history of conversion symptoms; evidence of past or current depression or of psychosis; difficulty in confirming a diagnosis of either angina pectoris or Prinzmetal's angina; evidence of legal or financial remuneration for disability; evidence of significant secondary gain, such as relief from work or other responsibilities; and/or evidence that the patient does not foresee a substantially improved postsurgical existence for himself. These signs should give clinicians pause before proceeding with cardiac surgery. Equally important, psychodiagnostic and psychotherapeutic input should be sought early. For example, the routine, team-member involvement of a psychiatrist on CCU and cardiac surgery staffs has been urged for years by many clinicians but has not been widely adopted in practice. Such early, regular involvement should allow the presentation of the consulting psychotherapist as routine, rather than seeming to be prompted by the physician's belief that the patient is crazy or phony. A benign early beginning, then, allows the psychotherapist to convey to the chronic pain patient, in word and deed, that he will remain available to the patient on a long-term basis, that he will not abandon him, regardless of fluctuations in pain and regardless of "failure" on the patient's part to "improve."

With both angina and pseudoangina patients who have suffered MIs, the scope of the therapist's task is greatly expanded. Here the therapist and patient are no longer dealing only with pain and the *threat* of damage or death, but with real, often catastrophic, damage. Thus, the real and symbolic consequences of the infarct must enter into the treatment plan. For example, the multiple changes in economic capacity, family role, and physical capacity must be addressed, as must the pos-

sible symbolic meanings of infarction: castration or regression
to child or invalid status. Concrete behavioral changes, ade-
quacy of comprehension of the anatomical pathology and
pathophysiology involved, and related issues must be focused
on. In fact, post-MI psychotherapeutic intervention is itself a
broad field of clinical and scientific endeavor with its own large
literature. Summaries of this literature are provided by Razin
(1982, 1984a).

With angina and pseudoangina patients, especially when
there has been an MI, one must not lose sight of the frequent
problem of noncompliance—for example, with exercise, medication, and diet regimens. Baile and Engel (1978) and others have
provided a practical behavioral model for utilizing *self*-manage-
ment plans to reduce noncompliance in cardiac patients. Such
plans emphasize *patient* involvement in setting goals and steps
in rehabilitation, and one of the consulting psychotherapist's
most valuable contributions to his internist consultees may lie
in his helping the internist to devise and implement such strategies.

Since there is substantial evidence of heightened physiological reactivity in CAD patients, the use of somatic interventions should be considered. Progressive relaxation or biofeedback training may help lower heart rate (HR) but is even more
likely to lower blood pressure (BP). Since heightened blood
pressure may be associated specifically with emotionally induced angina, relaxation and/or biofeedback training aimed at
BP may be of particular benefit. Beta-adrenergic blockers are, of
course, already in wide use for angina, several arrhythmias, hypertension, and general post-MI prophylaxis. Alpha blockers
may eventually prove to offer additional benefits, especially
where the angina is caused by coronary artery spasm. Until a
few years ago, only the relatively few Prinzmetal patients were
believed to have angina due to spasm, but more recently we
have come to realize that a much larger proportion of CAD patients suffer from some varying combination of spasm and
atherosclerosis. Antianxiety agents, such as the benzodiaze-
pines, should not be dismissed as either a trivial or dangerous
(because of tolerance effects) treatment—particularly if a rela-

tionship between anxiety and pain (or elevated HR or BP) can be demonstrated with a particular patient. In using antianxiety agents, one must closely monitor dosage range, duration of treatment, and the possibility of depression as a side effect. Nonetheless, medication may be useful, especially in the post-MI convalescent period.

Since angina pectoris patients may be more overtly anxious, "neurotic," histrionic, somatizing, or emotionally labile than nonanginal CAD patients, psychological interventions generally should be supportive, reassuring, but *not* necessarily symptom suppressive. Unlike many other (non-CAD) types of chronic pain, angina pectoris serves as a vital warning sign. Thus, interventions aimed at reducing this pain symptom without modifying its pathophysiology seem potentially risky. Angina pectoris patients may, however, benefit from biofeedback training aimed at HR and/or BP, as mentioned above.

Pseudoangina patients are psychogenically a quite heterogeneous group; that is, pseudoangina may develop as a manifestation of any of a variety of character disorders or psychiatric syndromes. It becomes crucial, then, whether working from a psychodynamic or a behavioral framework, to attempt to identify a specific underlying disorder, which should, in turn, suggest appropriate goals. Thus, for example, anxiety neurosis, panic disorder, chronic characterological depression, and endogenous depressive episodes might each present as pseudoangina, but each would have distinct treatment strategies and goals.

The range of psychiatric disturbance underlying pseudoangina probably extends further into the seriously or more chronically disturbed portion of the spectrum of psychiatric disturbances, including pan-neurotic character disorders, entrenched somatization disorders, and near psychotic or even frankly psychotic syndromes. It thus becomes even more important with these patients than with angina pectoris patients to adopt a supportive therapeutic stance: to avoid confronting defenses; to take a "commonsense," general practitioner stance; to place minimal emphasis on generating insights; to utilize the general principles of treating chronic (non-CAD) pain patients (outlined above) and even to expect that pain may relocate itself in some other organ system as therapy proceeds; and, of course, to avoid questioning the reality of the pain.

In certain instances, depending on the nature of the underlying syndrome, we may wish to suppress related symptoms. Thus, if "cardiac neurosis" seems to underlie the pseudo angina, hyperventilation might very usefully be approached via the didactic methods described above. Similarly, tachycardia may also respond to conditioning or biofeedback interventions. And, *unlike* angina pectoris, the primary (chest pain) symptom itself may warrant suppression, so that conditioning (either operant or classical) and suggestion (via hypnotherapy) may be usefully incorporated.

Antianxiety, antidepressant, or even antipsychotic medications may be indicated if specific underlying psychiatric disorders are delineated. Pseudoangina in the context of documented CAD, may, of course, complicate the use of antidepressants (and certain antipsychotics). One must be especially cautious about orthostatic hypotension, as well as preexistent and drug-induced conduction defects. (See Cassem, 1982, for an excellent recent review of cardiovascular effects of antidepressants.) But the widespread hesitation, especially among internists, to use antidepressants with virtually any cardiac patient is probably largely unwarranted (Glassman and Bigger, 1981).

In the relatively unusual instances where the patient in some way acknowledges psychic distress but does not realize that it may be related to his chest pain, a therapeutic focus on these problems may be feasible. Even in this instance, though, the emphasis should probably be largely supportive. In this context I have found it useful to deemphasize any relationship between psyche and soma, to acknowledge the chest pain as a real problem in its own right, and even to focus on it in detail. I then tell the patient that he may have to suffer with the chest pain for some time but that, in any case, he may wish to work on his (acknowledged) "emotional" problems, with which I may be able to help him. This approach attempts to meet the patient "where he is at," allows the patient to keep his symptoms, puts no pressure on him to view his physical symptoms as "psychosomatic," and may allow an eventually beneficial psychotherapeutic intervention to proceed.

With the great detail and number of these guidelines for managing pseudoangina, one might have an impression of prognostic optimism. These syndromes, however, tend to be chronic, pervasive, and resistant to treatment. Though the suggested interventions may be helpful with certain patients, psychotherapeutic intervention is generally not very potent in pseudoangina. It may be that concerted, creative, systematic efforts to devise and assess behavioral or multimodal (behavioral plus pharmacological) interventions will yield more reason to be optimistic, but such optimism must await the appearance and systematic assessment of these newer interventions.

Conclusions and Directions for Research

Coronary artery disease is clearly a very common, very costly problem. It has been abundantly clear for more than a decade that several psychosocial factors are involved in the pathogenesis of CAD, either as predisposing or precipitating factors. And, while the precise identification of all these factors and assessment of their quantitative clinical significance still elude us, progress has been made recently, particularly in the area of Type A behavior. It is also clear that the impacts of CAD on psychosocial functioning are multiple and often severe.

The demonstration of psychosocial factors in the development of and recovery from CAD has raised the possibility of intervening psychologically—that is, reducing likely psychosocial "risk factors" in an attempt to prevent, ameliorate, or aid rehabilitation from CAD. From a seemingly "scientific" viewpoint, it might seem premature and inefficient to attempt to assess the effects of intervention when the "psychosocial risk factors" are still unclearly or controversially specified; however, the immensity of CAD as a public health problem lends urgency and legitimacy to such attempts, even in our current state of knowledge. Furthermore, as in other medical problems, elucidation of causes and mechanisms may follow from, rather than precede, such efforts.

Assessment of our own clinical work and that of other clinicians and researchers yields the following conclusions and recommendations.

Prevention. The CAD-prevention literature has been largely limited to the Type A behavior pattern. While there are major conceptual and empirical problems in the epidemiological, psychometric, and physiological TABP research, the pattern is clearly associated, though by unclear mechanisms, with increased CAD risk. Attempts to modify the TABP are thus of potentially great value. The handful of studies reporting such attempts offer suggestive evidence for the mutability of the TABP—most effectively, perhaps, by behavioral treatments. TABP intervention research, however, also suffers from conceptual and empirical problems (such as outcome criteria, measurement ambiguity, and subject selection). To address these problems, future TABP research should use *dynamic* physiological assessments, *secondary* prevention efforts, and multiple (behavioral, physiological, and self-report) outcome criteria.

Acute-Phase Intervention. Literature on intervention in this phase is best described as "lore": there is a rich, generally consistent, anecdotal literature on intervention and a small body of systematic research on patient experiences and reactions, but virtually no systematic study of the effects of acute-phase intervention. The pioneering work of Cassem and Hackett, and other psychiatric consultation-liaison groups, has made a substantial contribution in generating clinical descriptions and therapeutic guidelines, but, as Hackett himself indicates (1978), we must at this point apply more scientific methodology. Specifically, the prescriptive guidelines that emerge from the anecdotal literature need systematic assessment. No one has clearly demonstrated physiological improvement attributable to these interventions. In addition, the phenomenon of denial warrants more careful study, as do the acute-phase aspects of the TABP.

Convalescent/Rehabilitative-Phase Intervention. As in acute-phase intervention, our knowledge of this phase is largely informed by nonsystematic, often anecdotal reports. This body of literature is relatively substantial, reflective of a truly vast amount of cumulative clinical experience, and generally uniform (and consistent with our own clinical experience) in its recommendations (for example, that interventions be early, systematic, and educative and that social supports be mobilized). It is, however, largely unsupported by systematic study of intervention. And, as in the acute phase, while it might be tedious to test these recommendations singly, it would be quite valuable to test a number of them in "package" or comparative designs. Some of these now widely accepted recommendations (for example, for early mobilization and rehabilitative exercise) may not be well supported by controlled study.

The several studies of individual psychotherapeutic intervention, which vary widely in methodological rigor, suggest modest psychological and perhaps physiological gains as a result of *supportive* (versus exploratory) intervention. Behavioral interventions (including biofeedback and relaxation) may be effective with "cardiac neurotic" or "cardiac invalid" patients, though the evidence here is largely suggestive. Similarly, there is evidence that learning (instrumental and classical conditioning) may play an important role in the development of angina; and the possibility that behavioral intervention aimed at voluntary control of parameters will influence certain types of angina is intriguing, though as yet undemonstrated.

In clinical work with angina patients, not only behavioral but also psychodynamic and pharmacological interventions should be selected to target the individual patient's psychology and pathophysiology, though direct suppression of the angina itself is probably unwise. With pseudoangina patients the wide psychogenic diversity of the syndrome compels us to exert substantial effort to delineate a particular, presumably underlying, psychological mechanism or psychiatric syndrome. Such delineation should in most cases lead to formulation of specific treatment plans, which may differ substantially from each other, depending on the underlying psychiatric problem (for instance, a panic disorder might be treated quite differently from a somatization disorder). The impact of psychosocial interventions in pseudoangina is likely to be limited, at least in those cases where the pseudoangina seems to be part of an entrenched chronic character disorder. Nonetheless, in many instances behavioral or somatic interventions may effectively reduce the primary (pain) symptom or related symptoms; or supportive intervention may alleviate some of the psychic suffering, if not the psychopathology. However, since angina and (even more so) pseudoangina are psychophysiological phenomena that are virtually unexamined by systematic research, efforts to delineate the complex psychophysiologies of these syndromes (for instance, their comparability to other pain syndromes) are as much needed as are studies of clinical intervention.

Group interventions are probably more appealing to MI patients, who characteristically show enthusiastic involvement and who clearly seem to benefit psychologically. Physiological benefits are less clear, although a few rigorous studies do suggest improved morbidity and mortality. Like the individual intervention literature, the group work stresses the need for supportive, concrete, didactic, nonexploratory approaches that do not resemble or bear the label of "psychotherapy."

In conclusion, the overall current status of psychosocial intervention in coronary disease is similar to that characterizing psychotherapy research about fifteen to twenty years ago (and still to some extent today): many clinicians practicing techniques and advocating theories that were much more lore than science, while debates ensued about whether "psychotherapy works." As psychotherapy researchers have refined *and tested* the questions (what kind of therapy, for what kind of patient, with which therapist, and under what circumstances, produces what kind of outcome), much greater precision and understanding, if not final answers, have begun to characterize the whole endeavor of psychotherapy research. Thus, in CAD psychosocial intervention, if we are to move from a "promising," controversial state of knowledge, we must move from the global clinical impression to the specific, tested hypothesis—especially in the acute and rehabilitative CAD (MI) phases, but also in the preventive phase.

While it is certainly our hope that this chapter (and this entire volume) provides clinicians with useful conceptual and clinical guidelines, it is also our hope that we have stimulated clinicians and researchers to test systematically the several hypotheses that this chapter has attempted to delineate.

References

Adsett, C. A., and Bruhn, J. G. "Short-Term Group Psychotherapy for Post-Myocardial Infarction Patients and Their Wives." *Canadian Medical Association Journal,* 1968, *99,* 577-584.

Baile, W. F., and Engel, B. T. "A Behavioral Strategy for Promoting Treatment Compliance Following Myocardial Infarction." *Psychosomatic Medicine,* 1978, *40,* 413-419.

Bartle, S. H., and Bishop, L. F. "Psychological Study of Patients with Coronary Heart Disease with Unexpectedly Long Survival and High Level Function." *Psychosomatics,* 1974, *15,* 68-69.

Bilodeau, C. B., and Hackett, T. P. "Issues Raised in a Group Setting by Patients Recovering from Myocardial Infarction." *American Journal of Psychiatry,* 1971, *128,* 73-78.

Blackburn, H. "Progress in the Epidemiology and Prevention of Coronary Heart Disease." In P. N. Yu and J. F. Goodwin (Eds.), *Progress in Cardiology.* Philadelphia: Lea & Febiger, 1974.

Blanchard, E. B., and Miller, S. T. "Psychological Treatment of Cardiovascular Disease." *Archives of General Psychiatry,* 1977, *34,* 1402-1413.

Bruhn, J. G., and others. "Patients' Reactions to Death in a Coronary Care Unit." *Journal of Psychosomatic Research,* 1970, *14,* 65-75.

Cassem, N. H. "Cardiovascular Effects of Antidepressants." *Journal of Clinical Psychiatry,* 1982, *43,* 22-29.

Cassem, N. H., and Hackett, T. P. "Psychiatric Consultation in a Coronary Care Unit." *Annals of Internal Medicine,* 1971, *75,* 9-14.

Cassem, N. H., and Hackett, T. P. "Psychological Rehabilitation of Myocardial Infarction Patients in the Acute Phase." *Heart and Lung,* 1973, *2,* 382-389.

Cassem, N. H., and Hackett, T. P. "Psychological Aspects of

Myocardial Infarction." *Medical Clinics of North America,* 1977, *61,* 711-721.

Cathey, C., and others. "The Relation of Life Stress to the Concentration of Serum Lipids in Patients with Coronary Artery Disease." *American Journal of the Medical Sciences,* 1962, *244,* 421-441.

Cooper, T., Detre, T., and Weiss, S. *Coronary-Prone Behavior and Coronary Heart Disease.* Washington, D.C.: National Heart, Lung, and Blood Institute, 1978.

Croog, S. M., Levine, S., and Lurie, Z. "The Heart Patient and the Recovery Process: A Review of the Literature on Social and Psychological Factors." *Social Science and Medicine,* 1968, *2,* 111-164.

Dembroski, T. M., and others. *The Type A Coronary-Prone Behavior Pattern: A Review.* Washington, D.C.: National Heart, Lung, and Blood Institute, 1980.

Doehrman, S. R. "Psycho-Social Aspects of Recovery from Coronary Heart Disease: A Review." *Social Science and Medicine,* 1977, *11,* 199-218.

Dominian, J., and Dobson, M. "Study of Patients' Psychological Attitudes to a Coronary Care Unit." *British Medical Journal,* 1969, *4,* 795-798.

Frank, K. A., Heller, S. S., and Kornfeld, D. S. "Psychological Intervention in Coronary Heart Disease." *General Hospital Psychiatry,* 1979, *1,* 18-23.

Friedman, M. *Pathogenesis of Coronary Artery Disease.* New York: McGraw-Hill, 1969.

Friedman, M. "The Type A Behavior Pattern: Some of Its Pathophysiological Components." *Bulletin of the New York Academy of Medicine,* 1977, *53,* 593-604.

Friedman, M., and others. "Feasibility of Altering Type A Behavior Pattern After Myocardial Infarction." *Circulation,* 1982, *66,* 83-92.

Garner, H. H., and Falk, M. A. "Recognizing the Patient with Pseudoangina." *Geriatrics,* 1970, *25,* 87-92.

Garrity, T. F. "Social Involvement and Activeness as Predictors of Morale Six Months After First Myocardial Infarction." *Social Science and Medicine,* 1973a, *7,* 199-207.

Garrity, T. F. "Vocational Adjustment After First Myocardial Infarction: Comparative Assessment of Several Variables Suggested in the Literature." *Social Science and Medicine,* 1973b, *7,* 705-715.

Glassman, A. M., and Bigger, J. T. "Cardiovascular Effects of Therapeutic Doses of Tricyclic Antidepressants." *Archives of General Psychiatry,* 1981, *38,* 815-820.

Granger, J. W. "Full Recovery from Myocardial Infarction: Psychological Factors." *Heart and Lung,* 1974, *3,* 600-610.

Groden, B. M., Allison, A., and Shaw, C. B. "Management of Myocardial Infarction: The Effect of Early Mobilization." *Scottish Medical Journal,* 1967, *12,* 435-446.

Groden, B. M., and Brown, R. I. F. "Differential Psychological Effects of Early and Late Mobilization After Myocardial Infarction." *Scandinavian Journal of Rehabilitation Medicine,* 1970, *2,* 60-86.

Gruen, W. "Effects of Brief Psychotherapy During the Hospitalization Period on the Recovery Process in Heart Attacks." *Journal of Consulting and Clinical Psychology,* 1975, *43,* 223-232.

Hackett, T. P. "The Use of Groups in the Rehabilitation of the Postcoronary Patient." *Advances in Cardiology,* 1978, *24,* 127-135.

Hackett, T. P., and Cassem, N. H. "Development of a Quantitative Rating Scale to Assess Denial." *Journal of Psychosomatic Research,* 1974, *18,* 93-100.

Hackett, T. P., Cassem, N. H., and Wishnie, H. A. "The Coronary Care Unit: An Appraisal of Its Psychological Hazards." *New England Journal of Medicine,* 1968, *279,* 1365-1370.

Haynes, S. G., and others. "The Relationship of Psychosocial Factors to Coronary Heart Disease in the Framingham Study." *American Journal of Epidemiology,* 1978, *107,* 362-381.

Helsing, K. J., Szklo, M., and Comstock, G. W. "Factors Associated with Mortality After Widowhood." *American Journal of Public Health,* 1981, *71,* 802-809.

Hurst, J. W., Logue, R. B., and Walter, P. F. "The Clinical Recognition and Management of Coronary Atherosclerotic Heart

Disease." In J. W. Hurst and others (Eds.), *The Heart.* (4th ed.) New York: McGraw-Hill, 1978.

Ibrahim, M. A., and others. "Management After Myocardial Infarction: A Controlled Trial of the Effect of Group Psychotherapy." *International Journal of Psychiatry in Medicine,* 1974, *5,* 253-268.

Jenkins, C. D. "Psychologic and Social Precursors of Coronary Disease." *New England Journal of Medicine,* 1971, *284,* 244-255, 307-317.

Jenkins, C. D. "The Coronary-Prone Personality." In W. D. Gentry and R. B. Williams, Jr. (Eds.), *Psychological Aspects of Myocardial Infarction and Coronary Care.* St. Louis: Mosby, 1975.

Jenkins, C. D. "Recent Evidence Supporting Psychologic and Social Risk Factors for Coronary Disease." *New England Journal of Medicine,* 1976, *294,* 987-997, 1033-1038.

Jenni, M. A., and Wollersheim, J. P. "Cognitive Therapy, Stress Management Training and Type A Behavior Pattern." *Cognitive Therapy and Research,* 1979, *3,* 61-73.

Kasl, S. V. "Social-Psychological Characteristics Associated with Behaviors Which Reduce Cardiovascular Risk." In A. J. Enelow and J. B. Henderson (Eds.), *Applying Behavioral Science to Cardiovascular Risk.* New York: American Heart Association, 1975.

Kimball, C. P. "Interviewing and Therapy in the Acute Situation." In T. B. Karasu and R. I. Steinmuller (Eds.), *Psychotherapeutics in Medicine.* New York: Grune & Stratton, 1978.

Klein, R. F., and others. "Transfer from a Coronary Care Unit." *Archives of Internal Medicine,* 1968, *122,* 104-108.

Kornfeld, D., Zimberg, S., and Malm, J. "Psychiatric Complications of Open-Heart Surgery." *New England Journal of Medicine,* 1965, *273,* 287-292.

Leigh, H., and others. "A Psychological Comparison of Patients in 'Open' and 'Closed' Coronary Care Units." *Journal of Psychosomatic Research,* 1972, *16,* 449-458.

Lenzner, A. S., and Aronson, A. L. "Psychiatric Vignettes from a Coronary Care Unit." *Psychosomatics,* 1972, *13,* 179-183.

Levenkron, J. C., and others. "Modifying the Type A Coronary-

Prone Behavior Pattern." *Journal of Consulting and Clinical Psychology*, 1983, *51*, 192-204.

Lynch, J. J. *The Broken Heart: The Medical Consequences of Loneliness*. New York: Basic Books, 1977.

Lynch, J. J., and others. "The Effects of Human Contact on Cardiac Arrhythmia in Coronary Care Patients." *Journal of Nervous and Mental Disease*, 1974, *158*, 83-99.

McAlister, A. L., and others. "Behavioral Science Applied to Cardiovascular Health: Progress and Research Needs in the Modification of Risk-Taking Habits in Adult Populations." *Health Education Monographs*, 1976, *4*, 45-74.

McGrath, F. J., and Robinson, J. C. "The Medical Social Worker in the Coronary Care Unit." *Medical Journal of Australia*, 1973, *2*, 1113-1118.

Matthews, K., and others. "Competitive Drive, Pattern A, and Coronary Heart Diseases: A Further Analysis of Some Data from the Western Collaborative Group Study." *Journal of Chronic Diseases*, 1977, *30*, 489-498.

Mills, M. E., and others. "Effect of Pulse Palpation on Cardiac Arrhythmia in Coronary Care Patients." *Nursing Research*, 1976, *25*, 378-382.

Mone, L. C. "Short-Term Psychotherapy with Postcardiac Patients." *International Journal of Group Psychotherapy*, 1970, *20*, 99-108.

Nagle, R., Gangola, R., and Picton-Robinson, I. "Factors Influencing Return to Work Following Myocardial Infarction." *Lancet*, 1971, *2*, 454-456.

Naismith, C. D., and others. "Psychological Rehabilitation After Myocardial Infarction." *British Medical Journal*, 1979, *1*, 439-442.

Prince, R., and Miranda, L. "Monitoring Life Stress to Prevent Recurrence of Coronary Heart Disease Episodes: Report of a Feasibility Study." *Canadian Psychiatric Association Journal*, 1977, *22*, 161-169.

Rahe, R. H. "Liaison Psychiatry on a Coronary Care Unit." *Journal of Human Stress*, 1975, *1*, 253-261.

Rahe, R. H., and others. "Group Therapy in the Out-Patient Management of Post-Myocardial Infarction Patients." *International Journal of Psychiatry in Medicine*, 1973, *4*, 77-88.

Rahe, R. H., and others. "Brief Group Therapy Following Myocardial Infarction: Eighteen Months Follow-Up of a Controlled Trial." *International Journal of Psychiatry in Medicine*, 1975, *6*, 349-358.

Rahe, R. H., and others. "Brief Group Therapy in Myocardial Infarction Rehabilitation: Three to Four Year Follow-Up of a Controlled Trial." *Psychosomatic Medicine*, 1979, *41*, 229-242.

Razin, A. M. "Psychosocial Intervention in Coronary Artery Disease: A Review." *Psychosomatic Medicine*, 1982, *44*, 363-387.

Razin, A. M. "Coronary Artery Disease." In H. B. Roback (Ed.), *Helping Patients and Their Families Cope with Medical Problems: A Guide to Therapeutic Group Work in Clinical Settings*. San Francisco: Jossey-Bass, 1984a.

Razin, A. M. "Psychotherapeutic Intervention in Angina. I: A Critical Review." *General Hospital Psychiatry*, 1984b, in press.

Razin, A. M. "Psychotherapeutic Intervention in Angina. II: Implications for Research and Practice." *General Hospital Psychiatry*, 1984c, in press.

Razin, A. M. "Type A Behavior: Can It Be Modified?" In L. Zohman and R. Kohn (Eds.), *Progress in Cardiac Rehabilitation*. New York: Thieme-Stratton, 1984d.

Rifkin, B. G. "The Treatment of Cardiac Neurosis Using Systematic Desensitization." *Behaviour Research and Therapy*, 1968, *6*, 239-241.

Rosenman, R. "The Role of Type A Behavior Pattern in the Pathogenesis of Ischemic Heart Disease, and Modifications for Prevention." *Advances in Cardiology*, 1978, *25*, 34-46.

Rosenman, R. H., and Chesney, M. A. "The Relationship of Type A Behavior Pattern to Coronary Heart Disease." *Activitas Nervosa Superior*, 1980, *22*, 1-45.

Rosenman, R. H., and others. "Coronary Heart Disease in the Western Collaborative Group Study: Final Follow-Up Experience of 8½ Years." *Journal of the American Medical Association*, 1975, *233*, 372-377.

Roskies, E. "Considerations in Developing a Treatment Program for the Coronary-Prone (Type A) Behavior Pattern." In P. O.

Davidson and S. M. Davidson (Eds.), *Behavioral Medicine: Changing Health Lifestyles.* New York: Brunner/Mazel, 1980.

Roskies, E., and others. "Changing the Coronary-Prone (Type A) Behavior Pattern in a Non-Clinical Population." *Journal of Behavioral Medicine,* 1978, *1,* 201-216.

Russek, H. I., and Russek, L. G. "Is Emotional Stress an Etiologic Factor in Coronary Heart Disase?" *Psychosomatic Medicine,* 1976, *38,* 63-67.

Soloff, P. H. "Denial and Rehabilitation of the Post-Infarction Patient." *International Journal of Psychiatry in Medicine,* 1978, *8,* 125-132.

Soloff, P. H. "Medically and Surgically Treated Coronary Patients in Cardiovascular Rehabilitation: A Comparative Study." *International Journal of Psychiatry in Medicine,* 1979, *9,* 93-106.

Stein, E. H., Murdaugh, J., and MacLeod, A., Jr. "Brief Psychotherapy of Psychiatric Reactions to Physical Illness." *American Journal of Psychiatry,* 1969, *125,* 1040-1047.

Thockloth, R. M., and others. "Is Cardiac Rehabilitation Really Necessary?" *Medical Journal of Australia,* 1973, *2,* 669-674.

Thompson, P. B. "Effectiveness of Relaxation Techniques in Reducing Anxiety and Stress Factors in Type A Post-Myocardial Infarction Patients." *Dissertation Abstracts,* 1977, *37A,* 5616-5617.

Thoresen, C. E., Telch, M. J., and Eagleston, E. R. "Approaches to Altering the Type A Behavior Pattern." *Psychosomatics,* 1981, *22,* 472-482.

Verwoerdt, A., and Dovenmuhle, R. H. "Heart Disease and Depression." *Geriatrics,* 1964, *19,* 856-863.

Weiner, H. J., Akabas, S. H., and Sommer, J. J. *Mental Health Care in the World of Work.* New York: Association Press, 1973.

Wheeler, E. D., and others. "Neurocirculatory Asthenia (Anxiety Neurosis, Effort Syndrome, Neurasthenia)." *Journal of the American Medical Association,* 1950, *142,* 878-889.

White, K. L., and others. "Angina Pectoris and Angina Innocens." *Psychosomatic Medicine,* 1955, *17,* 128-135.

Wickramasekera, I. "Heart Rate Feedback and the Management

of Cardiac Neurosis." *Journal of Abnormal Psychology,* 1974, *83,* 578-580.

Wishnie, H. A., Hackett, T. P., and Cassem, N. H. "Psychological Hazards of Convalescence Following Myocardial Infarction." *Journal of the American Medical Association,* 1971, *215,* 1292-1296.

Wynn, A. "Unwarranted Emotional Distress in Men with Ischaemic Heart Disease." *Medical Journal of Australia,* 1967, *2,* 847-851.

Name Index

195

Subject Index

A

Alpha blockers, and coronary artery disease, 179
Ambivalence, and surgery, 118
Ambulatory measures: for arrhythmia, 65, 71, 77-79, 104; for hypertension, 6-7
American Heart Association, 127
American Psychiatric Association, 72, 104, 124, 138, 146
Antianxiety agents, and coronary artery disease, 179-180, 181
Antidepressants, and coronary artery disease, 181
Antipsychotics: and arrhythmia, 69; and coronary artery disease, 181; and postoperative delirium, 135
Anxiety: and arrhythmia, 67-68, 72, 73, 96-99; and cardiac surgery, 137-138; and coronary artery disease, 160-161, 168, 180
Anxiolytics, and cardiac surgery, 138
Apresoline, in transactional psychophysiology, 42

Arrhythmias: ambulatory recording for, 65, 71, 77-79, 104; analysis of, 55-111; and anxiety, 67-68, 72, 73, 96-99; background on, 55-57; biofeedback for, 85-87, 88-91, 93-95, 96; case example of, 82-84, 102-103; classification of, 56-57; and clinical implications, 94-96; clinical interview for, 72-76; conclusions on, 103-104; and depression, 72, 73, 76, 79, 99-101; and ectopic beat, 61; and environmental demands, 70-71, 74-75; etiology and prevalence of, 64-67; evaluation of patient with, 71-84; factors exacerbating, 67-71; and family therapy, 92-93; and health risk profile, 80-82, 101-103; and hypnosis, 84, 88, 92, 94, 95; as impulse disturbance, treatment literature on, 93-94; mechanisms and pathophysiology underlying, 58-64; and meditation, 84, 91-92; and metabolic products, 64; as multiple consecutive ectopic

203